W9-AXX-950

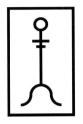

THE SIVANANDA COMPANION TO
MEDITATION

How to Master the Mind and Achieve Transcendence

THE SIVANANDA YOGA VEDANTA CENTER

A Fireside Book

Published by Simon & Schuster

New York   London   Toronto   Sydney   Singapore

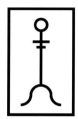

FIRESIDE
Rockefeller Center
1230 Avenue of the Americas
New York, NY 10020

Copyright © 2003 by Gaia Books Limited and Gaia Media
Text copyright © 2003 by The Sivananda Yoga Vedanta Center
All rights reserved,
including the right of reproduction
in whole or in part in any form.

FIRESIDE and colophon are registered trademarks
of Simon & Schuster, Inc

For information regarding special discounts for bulk purchases,
please contact Simon & Schuster Special Sales at 1-800-456-6798
or business@simonandschuster.com

Designed by Bridget Morley

Printed and bound in China by Imago

10 9 8 7 6 5 4 3 2 1

Library of Congress Cataloging-in-Publication data is available.

ISBN 0-7432-4611-X

CONTENTS

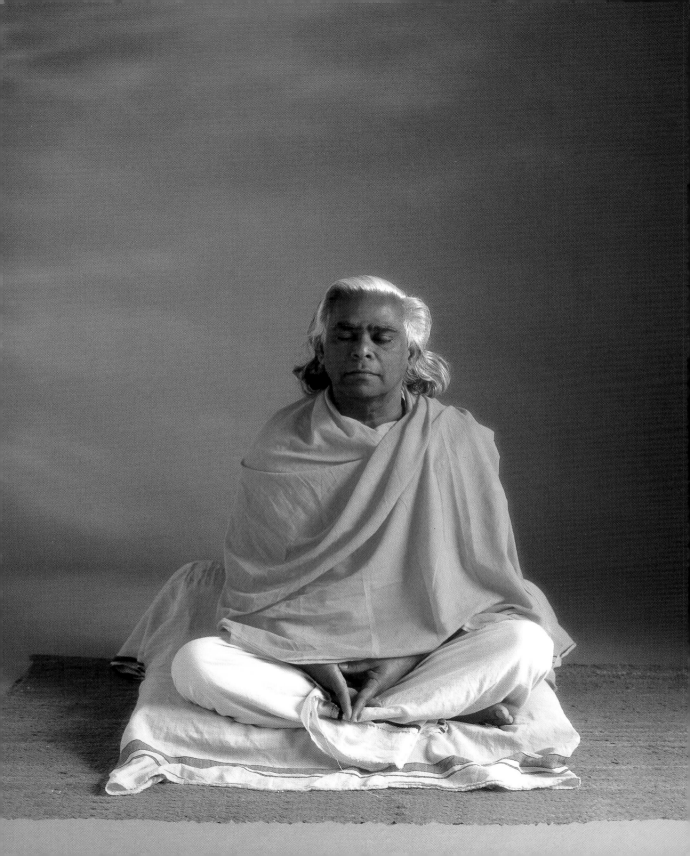

To Swami Vishnu-devananda
and to the Acharyas of the International Sivananda Yoga
Vedanta Centres (Executive Board Members)
for their support and encouragement in writing this book

*Through regular meditation, the mind
becomes clear and the motives pure.
The subconscious mind releases hidden
knowledge that allows a better understanding
of oneself and our relationship to the world.
The limited personality slowly dissolves
into an expanded consciousness.
Ultimately, the super-conscious or
intuitive forces are released,
leading to a life of wisdom and peace.*

SWAMI VISHNU-DEVANANDA

*Facing page: Swami Vishnu-devananda in meditation
Title page: dawn view of the lake at the Sivananda Yoga
Dhanwantari Ashram in Kerala, South India*

PREFACE

Meditation is at the core of the practice of yoga. It is both its main tool and its ultimate destination. This book presents a classical approach to the yogic path of meditation, which is called *raja yoga*. This knowledge dates from very ancient times and has been handed down from generation to generation through an unbroken lineage of teachers and students. The purpose of this book is to stimulate the reader's interest in the timeless practice of meditation and connect the reader with a time-tested spiritual tradition, probably the oldest one in the world.

The science of raja yoga is vast and complex. The knowledge in this book is based on the classical raja yoga tradition presented in the light of the direct experience of one of the great yoga masters of modern times, Swami Sivananda, and of one of his direct students, Swami Vishnu-devananda. Both of these teachers dedicated their lives to making yoga accessible to all. They present the intricate science of yoga in simple words, making it come alive through examples, stories, and anecdotes taken from daily life. They make it clear, straightforward, and resolutely practical. At the same time, they have never allowed the teachings to be diluted. Swami Vishnu-devananda, who was sent by his Master in the late 1950s to teach yoga to the West, fought all his life to preserve the purity and depth of the yogic knowledge he had received from his teacher in the Himalayas. A combination of simplicity and authenticity is the genius of these

two great teachers and explains the great success of their teachings in both the East and the West.

The following short account of the life's work of Swami Vishnu-devananda will hopefully convey the spirit in which he undertook the mission imparted to him by his teacher. In 1957 Swami Sivananda told him: "Go to the West. People are waiting." With this single instruction, a ten rupee note in his pocket, and no support other than his tremendous faith in his teacher and his indomitable willpower, Swami Vishnu-devananda left Swami Sivananda's *ashram* (retreat centre) in Rishikesh, North India, and started a long journey that took him to Sri Lanka, Indonesia, Japan, Hong Kong, and finally to the West. Everywhere he spread the knowledge of yoga, touching many people through his enthusiasm and boundless energy.

He arrived in San Francisco in the autumn of 1957 and explained to a suspicious immigration officer that he was coming to the United States of America to teach yoga. The official finally let him in after the young yogi had made an impressive demonstration of the full locust (an advanced yoga posture) on his desk! This was the beginning of a story that lasted thirty-five years, during which Swami Vishnu-devananda founded the Sivananda Yoga Vedanta Centre, one of the largest yoga organizations in the world

Group meditation at the Sivananda Yoga Dhanwantari Ashram in Kerala, South India. Group meditation confers a more powerful impact on the meditator than meditating alone.

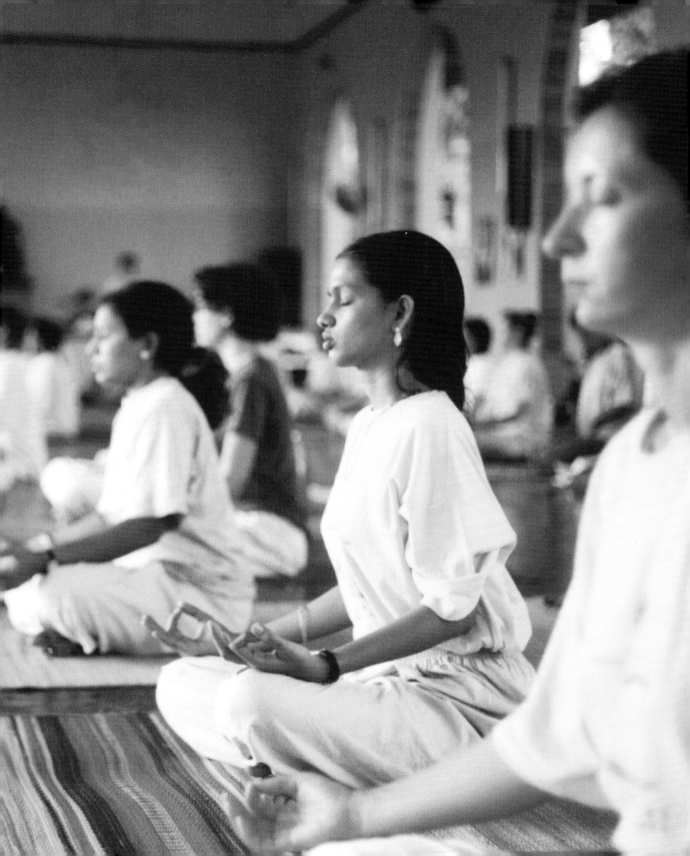

with over forty yoga centres and ashrams worldwide. In 1959 he wrote *The Complete Illustrated Book of Yoga*, which has sold over a million copies and remains a classic today. In 1969 he founded the True World Order, an international organization whose aim is to promote world peace and mutual understanding between nations, religions, and cultures. Swami Vishnu-devananda learned how to pilot a small plane and undertook numerous peace missions, flying over the world's trouble-spots at the risk of his life, dropping flowers and leaflets for peace over war zones and disputed borders. His peace flights took him to Belfast, Suez, and West Pakistan in 1971, and in 1983 he flew over the Berlin Wall from west to east.

In 1969 Swami Vishnu-devananda started the first yoga teachers' training course ever taught in the West. Since then, many thousands of teachers have been trained. In 1979 he wrote his second book *Meditation and Mantras*, aiming to "dispel the confusion that has arisen around the topic of meditation". Into this book he poured all his knowledge of the ancient science of meditation, mantras, and the four classical paths of yoga: *jnana yoga* (the yoga of knowledge), *bhakti yoga* (the yoga of universal love), *raja yoga* (the yoga of self-mastery), and *karma yoga* (the yoga of selfless action).

Swami Vishnu-devananda left his body in 1993 in India, after an extraordinary and eventful life lived for the total service of his mission: spreading the knowledge of yoga in the West and reviving it in its country of origin. The International Sivananda Yoga Vedanta Centres around the world continue his work and dedicate themselves to teaching yoga in the same spirit of purity and simplicity.

The Sivananda Yoga Vedanta Centres have been teaching meditation to beginners and advanced students for over thirty-five years. They have unrivalled experience in introducing this complex science to a public with a sincere interest in meditation but limited knowledge of traditional methods. As yoga has increased in popularity, the need has grown for a clear and simple book focusing specifically on the science of meditation.

The aim of this book is to present this science of meditation to those with little or no prior knowledge and to help them to get started in meditation practice. However, it does not present meditation as an isolated technique aiming at a quick fix for the stresses and strains of our daily lives, but rather as the central organ of a body of practices that constitute a way of life. The challenge in writing this book was to present the practice of meditation as a simple and effective method to regain inner and outer harmony. At the same time the reader's attention is gently draw to the fact that success in meditation will be in direct proportion to the effort expended in preparing for the practice.

It is not the purpose of this book to elaborate on the deep philosophy that underlies the practice of meditation. The more advanced practitioner can refer to Swami Vishnu-devananda's book *Meditation and Mantras*, available at Sivananda Yoga Vedanta Centres (see page 152).

HOW TO USE THIS BOOK

We recommend that you look through the whole book first for an overview of the process involved. Beginning a new meaningful activity is always exciting. Start by creating a sacred space for your practice. Use your creativity to make it simple but beautiful, so that it is a joy to sit there for your daily practice.

Make a resolve to try the practice of meditation for six months. Fix a time for your daily practice and make a strong resolve to stick to it. Start with the sense of an exciting new adventure: you are about to embark on the most fascinating and challenging of all journeys: one that will bring you back to your true Self. So celebrate and be grateful that this desire and inspiration has come to you. It is a blessing to be motivated to uplift one's life and expand one's awareness.

Keep a spiritual diary to record your progress: note how long you meditated, the quality of your concentration, the thoughts that troubled you the most, and what other challenges you met.

After a few months of practice, reflect and see what changes meditation has brought about in your life. Re-read Chapter Two, The Yogic Lifestyle, and think of what other positive changes you could make in your life: maybe an improvement in your diet, less time watching TV, getting up a little earlier, doing regular exercise, or spending more time in nature.

Once you have settled in your practice you can move on to the advanced part of the book. Reflect on Chapter Eight, The Art of Right Living, and revisit Chapter Four, The Art of Positive Thinking. You will grow aware that a change in personality comes from a shift in consciousness, not from a mere change of surroundings. Reflect on the necessity of uplifting the level of your thoughts.

At this point in your practice, you will probably feel the need for direct guidance from a teacher. Becoming aware of one's mental habits is a challenging task. Invoking within oneself enough humility, courage, and determination to overcome them requires guidance and encouragement from an experienced practitioner.

Always remember Swami Sivananda's "triple secret formula" for success in yoga and meditation: "Practise, practise and... practise!"

If this book can stimulate your interest for the inner quest and get you started on your path, it will have reached its goal.

We wish you strength, inspiration, and joy on your journey. May the blessings of the ancient and modern yogis be with you!

THE SIVANANDA YOGA VEDANTA CENTRE

INTRODUCTION

The science of meditation is a universal tradition that traces its origin to thousands of years before the advent of today's civilization, surviving unchanged as it has passed from generation to generation. It has endured in its original form because within its simple framework lie the principal teachings and approaches that make up the substance of all known philosophies, religions, and disciplines. Meditation is by definition transcendental, a word used to convey the beauty of the practice, in which all fears, desires, longings, and negative emotions are left behind.

Many people come to meditation, not because they want to hide in a cave in the Himalayas withdrawing from the mainstream, but because they feel unfulfilled and empty, with stress, anxiety, frustration, and depression playing a much larger part in their lives than they would like. They realize there is a restlessness and dissatisfaction in their daily life and they have a vague notion that their search for happiness, peace, and contentment requires a different approach than that offered by Western society. They may be unsure of what meditation can do, but know it promises relief from the high tension and roller-coaster speed of today's technology-led culture.

Meditation gives this relief and much more. It teaches us that there is a power within each one of us, an energy, a peace, and a wisdom, which we can tap into once we know it is available. This power inspires, encourages, reinforces, and gives strength to those who seek to grow in a positive direction. You may be unaware of this inner resource, or have misconceptions about it. You may be like the Indian farmer who moved to a house in the city and lived in darkness because he did not know what those strange boxes in the wall could do. The power, the light is there and available to all; we need only to connect ourselves with the current. This source of wisdom is the *Self*. The Self is not the individual body or mind, but that aspect deep inside each person that knows the truth. It exists in each being and yet it exists independently also. Some call it Cosmic Consciousness, Holy Spirit, Universal Mind, Love, the Peace that Passeth all Understanding, the Absolute; others call it Buddha, Christ, Allah, Brahman, God.... The names and paths are many, but there is one supreme essence that pervades all of life. This Self is impossible to understand with our minds. There is no way to intellectually define or describe that which is limitless. Only through direct experience can this essence be known. Through the protracted practice of meditation we can still the outgoing mind, develop intuitive abilities, and touch that part of the supreme essence that lies within all; a process which brings peace, compassion, joy, and understanding in its wake. Yoga likens the mind to a lake, with the ripples on the lake representing our thoughts and emotions. When the ripples subside the lake is still and we can see the precious jewels lying silently in their glory at the bottom.

The first lesson that we learn when we start the process of meditation – for process it is – is to look into our own minds. To many this may seem a difficult task. Western psychology teaches us to look at how other people think and behave in order to gain insight into our own minds. However, the tradition of yoga states clearly that we must leave other people's lives alone and focus only on ourselves. Yoga teaches that to find peace we must first develop peace within ourselves. The challenge is to gain control of our own personal internal world.

When we look within, what do we find? We find a mind constantly conversing with itself, jumping from one thought or emotion to the next, caught in continual motion, running away from this or running towards that, robbing us of the ability to focus and be still. We are looking for peace but our search leads us mistakenly to look outside and we find ourselves resorting to drugs, alcohol, cigarettes, television, overeating, oversleeping, or overworking in the hope of stilling the mind. We unconsciously lead ourselves into a never-ending cycle of desire, further than ever from our goal of peace.

Meditation is the art of slowing down and focusing the mind; the seventh step of the eight-step path of yoga known as *raja yoga*, which aims at complete mastery over body and mind. Meditation (*dhyana* in Sanskrit) is a state of consciousness and as such is difficult to describe. The great *rishis* or sages from India compare the state of mind in meditation to the uninterrupted flow of oil from one vessel into another. There is movement, but it is the movement of the natural flow of consciousness with no interruption from the thoughts and desires that normally crowd our minds. It is not a void, as is commonly conceived, but the fullness of pure consciousness itself, the substratum behind the mind and the ground of all existence. With the stilling of the mind comes the realization that we have within ourselves that which we were fruitlessly seeking outside – selfless love; the very source of bliss. Swami Sivananda tells us that this natural state is our birthright, which we have mislaid through misguided actions and thought patterns. To find again our true nature we need to realign ourselves to the eternal, universal laws of health and harmony in order to create the conditions in which we can practise the art of meditation.

This realignment requires a knowledge of how our thought processes work and what we need to be able to meditate. Much has been said and written about meditation, yet it takes years to understand its nature. It cannot be taught, just as sleep cannot be taught. We may have a comfortable mattress, a warm room, and no disturbances, but sleep may not come. Sleep itself is not in anyone's hands. We just fall into it. In the same way, meditation comes by itself, but only when the mind is still. To acquire this stillness of mind requires daily practice as it does not come automatically. Once we have learned how to concentrate or focus the mind for a time, quietening the thought waves, the conditions will be right and we fall effortlessly into the meditative state. The sixth step in the raja yoga system is known as *dharana*, concentration, and the sages spend much time explaining how the practice of concentration is an essential prerequisite to the practice of meditation.

When we start to meditate most of us have serious difficulty focusing our mind and keeping it positive. We may suffer from depression or feel burnt-out from an unbalanced lifestyle. So in the beginning we need to direct our efforts towards pulling ourselves slowly out of this negative state. We start to readjust the way we live, allowing the nervous system to calm down and gradually, over time, developing a clear, positive goal for life. This way we start to regain control over our mind, and gradually develop the ability consciously to gather in its rays and focus them on a single positive thought.

This book is intended to guide us away from unhealthy and unrewarding states of mind to one that is full, profound, and joyful. The journey is long and has challenges that require patience, perseverance, and tenacity.

We are at first not fully aware of the inner resistance to change, which is deeply rooted in one part of our mind. It is only when we start clearing up that we realize how cluttered a room can be and it is the same with the mind. We may not see the thick layer of dust that has accumulated within; so when we start, doubt may creep in. This doubt is a trick of the mind to make us stop the practice and return to a state of unawareness, but we are advised by the masters to take no notice. They urge us to continue with redoubled energy – meditation has to become an integral part of life, as basic to life as food and sleep. They entreat us to trust their promise that it is possible to train the mind to gather its energy, turning it within to illumine the deeper part of the Self and reach the full awareness of ourselves and the meaning of our life. Meditation will take us to a state of the awareness of our true being, a state of complete and spontaneous relaxation, innocence, and bliss.

STARTING OUT

CHAPTER ONE

THE PRACTICE OF MEDITATION –
A TWELVE-STEP GUIDE

Swami Vishnu-devananda would say, as mentioned in our introduction, that it is not possible to teach someone how to meditate, any more than it is possible to teach them how to sleep. Sleep overtakes us only when we detach our mind from its concerns. Meditation also cannot be forced, but unlike sleep, it is a conscious state. We need a degree of willpower to remain in the state of heightened awareness that occurs when we meditate. However, at the same time we need to relax, letting go of all expectations and desires. This subtle balance between the effort needed to sustain concentration on the one side and detachment from all distractions on the other is the art of meditation. We learn to focus the mind without struggle, yet maintain enough control to avoid a drift into reverie.

To attain this state of relaxed awareness we need to prepare ourselves, and there are several steps that will help us. It is important to reiterate that meditation is a process and, as such, takes time. Be gentle and patient with your mind; do not expect miracles. The more care and attention you give to the preparation, the more positive the results.

I THE PLACE

It is best to have a special room for meditation, but if this is impossible, as it is for most of us, try to separate off a portion of a room, reserving it solely for your practice if you can. Maintain it as a space to be used only for meditation, clean and tidy, free from distracting vibrations and associations, and allow only those who respect its sacredness to enter.

The place of focus

Set up a little table as the focal point of the room, with a candle or, better still, a small oil lamp, light being a potent spiritual symbol.

Wearing a meditation shawl made of cotton or wool and sitting on a simple rug or mat will reinforce the calm atmosphere around you when you sit for meditation.

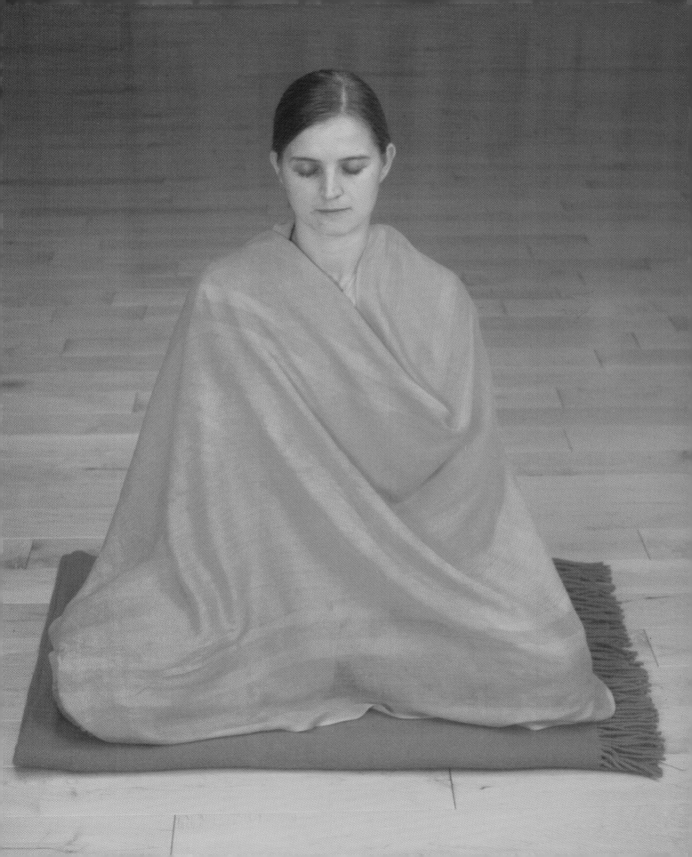

Gazing at the steady flame before you start your meditation practice will bring concentration and introversion of the mind. This gazing is actually a concentration exercise in its own right, as explained on pages 63–5. A flower or vase of flowers will enhance the atmosphere and fill the mind with joy. Burning incense in the morning and evening has a strongly purifying effect on the energy of the space. Use natural (not chemical) incense such as sandalwood, with its calming and cooling effect on the mind, or fragrances such as rose or frankincense.

If you are of a religious nature, set up an image of an uplifting spiritual symbol, such as the OM symbol, the Cross, or the Star of David; or a picture of Christ, Krishna, the Divine Mother, or Buddha. Choose what speaks to your heart and soul and helps your mind to turn within, away from worldly concerns. The powerful vibrations from repeated meditation practice will remain in the room, creating a magnetic aura, and within six months the peace and purity of the atmosphere will be quite tangible. In times of stress you can sit in the space, practise for half an hour, and experience great comfort and relief.

Purifying the meditation area

For more advanced meditators we recommend a practice called *arati* (see page 105).

Which direction to face

Sitting on a clean mat (a folded woollen blanket or cotton mat are excellent for this) in front of the table, face north or east to take advantage of favourable magnetic vibrations. These directions are considered to be the most conducive to spiritual concentration.

Meditating in nature

It scarcely needs mentioning that natural environments are much more favourable to the practice of meditation than cities, where pollution from noise, traffic, electronic machinery, and the high stress levels of many of the people around can make it difficult to

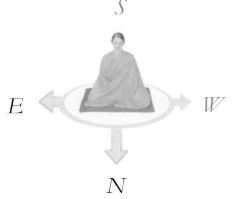

Face north or east to take advantage of favourable magnetic vibrations.

Swami Sivananda in meditation

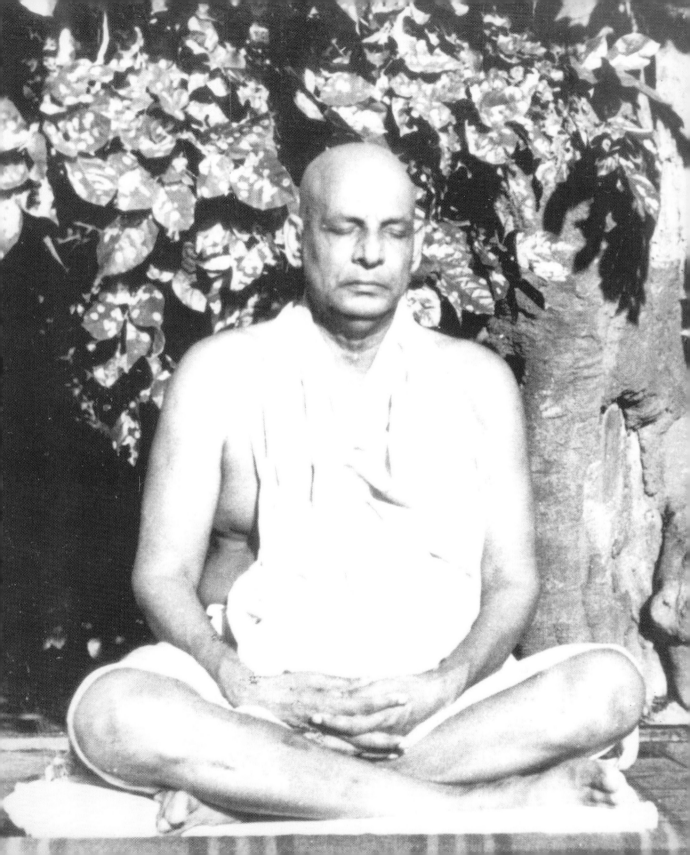

concentrate. If you can, try to take advantage of any opportunity to meditate in nature – on a beach facing the ocean, on a peaceful river bank, under a tree, on a mountain, with the rising or setting sun. You will find the meditation qualitatively different. If, like most of us, you have to meditate in the city, you can still create a protected and sacred environment and it is certainly better to meditate in a city than not to meditate at all!

2 THE TIME

The most effective times for the practice of meditation are at dawn and dusk, when the atmosphere is charged with special spiritual force. The most desirable time is *brahmamuhurta*, the hours between four and six a.m. In these quiet hours after sleep, the mind and atmosphere are clear and unruffled by activities of the day. Refreshed and free of worldly concerns, concentration comes without effort. If this is not feasible, choose a time when you can retreat from daily activities and calm your mind. In the evening around sunset is also a good time or just before going to bed. With the mind freed from the tensions accumulated during the day and tuned to a higher state, you will quickly fall into deep sleep after meditating. At whatever time you choose, make sure you know you will not be disturbed by outside distractions.

3 THE HABIT

It is important that you maintain consistency in your practice as well as meditating at the same time each day. The subconscious mind needs regularity to develop the habit of settling down and focusing easily. Start with fifteen to twenty minutes' daily practice and gradually build up to an hour. If you can't manage this, aim for thirty minutes daily. It is better to meditate every day for thirty minutes than once a week for two hours.

Even when you travel, meditate every day. As you establish the practice, you will actually feel the need to meditate every morning; if circumstances prevent you from practising, you will experience an

At dawn the atmosphere is charged with a special spiritual force, making this an ideal time to meditate.

inner discomfort, similar to how you feel if you start your day without washing. You will realize that meditation is a mental cleansing, necessary for mental wellbeing. You will find you do not want to miss even a single day of practice.

4 THE SITTING POSITION

Sit in a comfortable steady posture, with spine and neck erect but not tense. The psychic current needs to travel unimpeded from the base of the spine to the top of the head, helping to steady the mind and encourage concentration. A comfortable cross-legged posture provides a firm base for the body, but it is not necessary to place the legs in *padmasana*, the classic lotus posture. You may wish to sit in *siddhasana*, the half-lotus position, or in any simple cross-legged position. Sitting on a cushion will help the thighs relax and bring the knees closer to the ground. In these sitting positions, a triangular path is created for the flow of energy, containing it rather than allowing it to disperse in all directions. Metabolism and breathing slow down as concentration deepens.

Elderly or less able people may wish to sit on a comfortable chair, with ankles crossed. Lying down is not recommended because you relax completely and may find it almost impossible to ward off sleep. The mild muscular contraction necessary to hold the back upright in a sitting position keeps you alert. Try to relax the rest of the body as much as possible, especially the muscles of the face, neck, and shoulders. The chest should be open, with the rib cage lifted to encourage abdominal breathing.

There are various possible positions for the hands:

1 Placed on your knees in the *chin-mudra* position

2 The right hand cupped in the left, with palms turned upwards

3 Hands clasped loosely by interlocking the fingers.

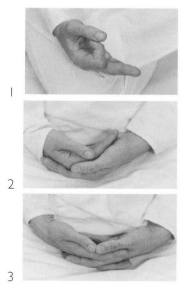

1

2

3

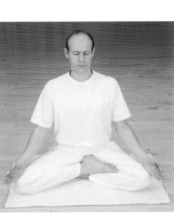

Siddhasana, the half-lotus position

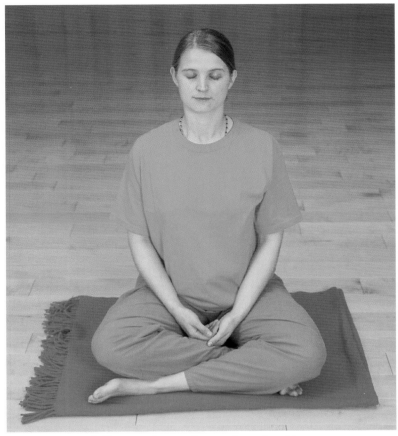

Sukhasana, the simple cross-legged position

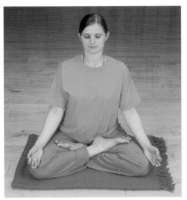

Padmasana, the full lotus position

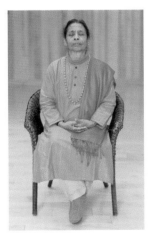

Sitting in a chair, keep your spine straight and your ankles crossed.

Initially you may find it difficult to keep the back straight for more than a few minutes. The practice of *asanas* (yoga postures) for as little as thirty minutes a day will strengthen your back, making it easy for you to sit comfortably over a long period of time. The actual purpose of asanas, according to the classical texts, is to be able to sit effortlessly and without fatigue for prolonged stretches. Patanjali, author of the most significant treatise on raja yoga, says that the meditation pose should be *"sukham sthiram"*, pleasant and firm. Swami Sivananda says one should feel as steady as a mountain outwardly and as flowing as honey within.

Your body will be at ease and will require no attention; a little like a vehicle that has been parked and can be forgotten about. You will be able to disconnect from the sense of being the body and focus on the deeper aspects of consciousness. It may take a few months to master the meditation posture; however, the confidence and satisfaction gained from training the body is well worth striving for. This first achievement in your practice will give you much joy and the confidence to meet greater challenges.

5 THE BREATH

Consciously try to relax and make the breath rhythmic. Begin with one minute of deep abdominal breathing to bring oxygen to the brain. Then, slowing the breath down to an imperceptible rate, inhale and exhale rhythmically, for approximately three seconds each. The breath becomes light and completely silent. This technique is a *pranayama* (breath control) exercise that steadies the *prana* (breath) and thereby quietens the mind. For more on pranayama see page 39.

6 THE MIND

For your meditation practice to succeed, it is important to transform the suffering and negativity of the mind by welcoming heightened awareness, broad vision, joy, and contentment into your life. The degree to which you are successful in your practice will be in direct proportion to your commitment to this goal. There must be an earnest desire to refrain from "sleeping with open eyes", as Swami Vishnu-devananda would say. Our minds love ease; we love to be on holiday, doing what we want when we want, with no sense of responsibility. We feel free with all options in our life possible. However, these options remain only potentialities, mere dreams, and without effort nothing in our lives changes. For real change to occur we need to understand that commitment is not a limitation of freedom, but, on the contrary, an assertion of the freedom to choose the direction in which we want our lives to go.

RAJA YOGA

The system of raja yoga, one of the four great paths of yoga, was first compiled by the great sage Patanjali Maharishi nearly 2,000 years ago in a series of sutras or aphorisms known as the *Raja Yoga Sutras*. Raja yoga is a scientific system that aims at disciplining the mind, body, and senses in order to attain complete control of the mind. Timeless and profound, its philosophy and psychological insights take the individual step by step through deep changes. The path consists of eight steps: *yamas* (abstentions), *niyamas* (observances), *asanas* (postures), *pranayama* (control of breath), *pratyahara* (withdrawal of the senses), *dharana* (concentration), *dhyana* (meditation), and *samadhi* (the superconscious state). The yamas and niyamas purify and uplift the mind. Asanas and pranayama strengthen the body and help towards control of the mind. The practice of pratyahara curbs the outgoing nature of the mind and conserves energy. Dharana leads to a quietening of the mind, dhyana to inner peace, and samadhi to transcendental or super-consciousness. The practice of meditation is central to the attainment of its goal.

The commitment we need to make is to live in the present moment, to give up living in the past, daydreaming or worrying about an imaginary future. In short it means controlling the tendency we all have to live in a fantasy world, a world in which we use the imagination to create a defence against suffering. Meditation allows us to see things as they are, without the masking veil of our likes and dislikes, without fear or hope. Start every meditation session asserting this willingness to face reality without escaping into imagination. It is not easy to do this, and initially you may try to take refuge in familiar defence strategies. But be patient, and over a period of time, gently coax the mind away from these destructive thought patterns. Gradually you will grow aware that you need to stop escaping into distraction whenever difficulties arise. Detachment from hopes and fears protects against suffering. By making the commitment to your wellbeing at each and every practice session, by gently commanding the mind to be quiet for a specific length of time, by focusing only on the present moment, your life will be immeasurably enhanced.

7 CHOOSING A POINT OF CONCENTRATION

Try to select a focal point on which the mind can rest. The mind needs a point of anchorage to ground itself as it usually spends much of the time daydreaming, disconnected from the present moment. This is partly achieved by bringing the awareness to the posture and the breath. But it can be further strengthened by bringing the attention to a specific point in the body. There are energy points in the body that are particularly appropriate and helpful to focus upon. These points are called *chakras*, or energy centres. This knowledge belongs to a branch of yoga called *kundalini yoga*, a specialized branch of the path of raja yoga. Kundalini yoga focuses on these energy centres in order to release the energy stored in them and bring about an expansion of consciousness. There are seven major chakras in the body and many more secondary ones. They are located in the *astral body* (a body of energy that is like a subtle etheric double of the physical body),

along the spinal column. They correspond to the different levels of consciousness, or the different levels of expression of our inner energies. The three lower chakras correspond to the more basic desires of the mind, the desire for security, for pleasure and for the expression of our individuality. The fourth, the heart chakra, corresponds to the expression of our energy as love; the fifth, the throat chakra, is the centre where consciousness expands to encompass knowledge of past and future incarnations. The sixth energy centre, located at the point between the eyebrows, is the centre for intuitional knowledge. The last, on the top of the head, corresponds to a state of union with cosmic consciousness.

Swami Sivananda recommends that we focus either on the heart centre (*anahata chakra*) or the centre between the eyebrows (*ajna chakra*). According to the science of kundalini yoga, one can meditate on any one of the chakras. However, the masters warn us that we must be ready for the energy release that is produced if we do so. Energy of course is neutral, and will empower whatever it is with which we identify. If the mind still strongly identifies with the instinctive desires, the newly released energy will feed these desires, strengthening them, and preventing us from bringing our awareness to higher states of consciousness. Until the mind is thoroughly purified, it is safer to focus on the higher chakras.

Swami Vishnu-devananda advises people with a more emotional type of personality to focus on the heart centre. This centre is ideal for those who find it easy to relate to others and the world at large through their feelings. They will find it easy to invoke devotion to an ideal, since this part of their personality is already active. Focusing on the heart centre will help to channel emotional energy and allow it to manifest as selfless love. The heart will expand.

If your personality is predominantly intellectual – if you tend to trust your thoughts more often than your feelings – you will find it easier to focus on the point between the eyebrows. This is the centre for self-awareness. Focusing on this centre will uplift the intellect and

KUNDALINI YOGA

The astral body
Every organism has an astral body, a subtle body through which the vital energy or prana of the body flows. It corresponds closely to the physical body and houses the senses and the emotional, mental, and intellectual faculties including the subconscious mind and prana. The physical body proceeds from the astral body, and the two bodies are connected by means of a subtle cord along which the vital currents pass. At the time of death this cord is severed and the astral and physical bodies separate.

Kundalini
Kundalini is a primordial cosmic power, a psychic spiritual force that lies dormant in the astral body of every human being. When awakened through various yoga practices, kundalini leads to the state of supreme consciousness or spiritual enlightenment. Through the sustained practice of kundalini yoga under the guidance of a guru, the advanced student acquires a thorough knowledge of the astral body and its structure as well as purification of both the physical and astral bodies. The aspirant "awakens" the kundalini by disciplining the body, purifying the nadis (see right), and controlling the prana through pranayama (see page 39). Once aroused, kundalini energy is pulled upward through the chakras (the psychic centres of the body – see right), until it reaches the chakra at the top of the head, where spiritual enlightenment occurs.

Each of the seven chakras has its own geometric form, sound vibration, colour, function, element, presiding deity, and mystic vibration, and during meditation is visualized as a lotus with a specific number of petals.

The nadis

Nadis are channels in the astral body through which the vital force, the prana, flows. According to yogic theory, there are around 72,000 nadis – known as meridians in the Chinese system – which correspond to the nerves in the physical body. The most important of these is the *sushumna*, the astral body's counterpart to the spinal cord. On either side of it are two nadis known as *ida* and *pingala*, which correspond to the left and right sympathetic cords in the physical body. With the kundalini practices the idea is for the aspirant to bring the flow of prana away from the ida and pingala into the sushumna, awakening the kundalini and allowing it to rise.

The chakras

The seven major chakras (literally "wheel" in Sanksrit) are subtle centres of vital energy and consciousness in the astral body. The major nerve plexuses are their counterparts in the physical body. These centres remain inactive in most people. However, in kundalini yoga the energy is consciously moved gradually through the sushumna nadi (see left) and passes through each chakra, where latent psychic powers are awakened and, as a result, different states of consciousness are experienced. Each chakra expresses a particular level of evolution of consciousness.

The location of the chakras and their corresponding centres in the physical body are:

1 Muladhara – at the lower end of the spinal column, corresponding to the sacral plexus
2 Swadhisthana – in the region of the genital organs, corresponding to the prostatic plexus
3 Manipura – at the navel, corresponding to the solar plexus
4 Anahata – at the heart, corresponding to the cardiac plexus
5 Vishuddha – in the throat region, corresponding to the laryngeal plexus
6 Ajna – in the region between the eyebrows, corresponding to the cavernous plexus
7 Sahasrara – at the crown of the head, corresponding to the pineal gland.

will gradually free it from its narrow and selfish vision. Eventually the doors of intuition will open and you will perceive reality without the limited screen of the intellect. This state is often referred to as the opening of the third eye.

Obviously everyone has both an emotional and an intellectual side to their personality, but one aspect is usually predominant. Neither point is better than the other. Concentrating on either of these points will lead to the same result: an expansion of consciousness. The main purpose here is to train your energy to stabilize on one point. Once you have chosen a point, keep to it for the rest of your life. If you change, the energy will become unsteady again, which will make the mind wander. The mind consists of energy. The energy has to be trained to flow in a harmonious way. You cannot stop the energy from flowing, but you want the flow to be steady and quiet, like pouring oil from one vessel to another, so that you feel no movement and the flow is uninterrupted.

Try not to confine your mind when you focus on your chosen energy centre. This may seem paradoxical, but focusing is a springboard for concentration, allowing the mind to expand into infinite space. Meditation is not merely an act of will, but more a commitment of the heart. Where your heart goes, your mind goes, and where your mind goes, your life will follow.

8 CHOOSING AN OBJECT OF CONCENTRATION

You will find that you need to stabilize your mental energy even further. The mind now needs to be trained in the art of concentration itself and for this you need to give your mind an object on which to focus. All previous steps are actually a preparation for this purpose – keeping the mind on a single object for more than a few seconds. Concentration is supported by a firm posture, a quietened breath, and focus on an energy centre. This is still not meditation. Meditation is a state beyond concentration, which is reached only once the mind is perfectly concentrated.

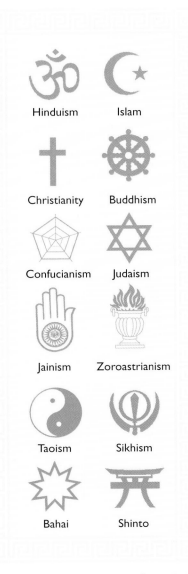

Hinduism   Islam

Christianity   Buddhism

Confucianism   Judaism

Jainism   Zoroastrianism

Taoism   Sikhism

Bahai   Shinto

The major world religions have their own symbols, any of which can provide a potent focus for meditation.

Yoga considers the use of *mantras* (words of power) as an essential tool for concentration (see Chapter Five). The practice is simple: repeat the mantra mentally and synchronize this repetition with your breath. It will help if you can feel the vibration of the mantra emanating from your concentration centre. The breath, the concentration centre, and the sound of the mantra become one point. However, the mantra can also be repeated out loud, especially if you are becoming drowsy. You can also start the practice by repeating the mantra aloud, gradually lowering your voice to a whisper, then reducing it to the most powerful method, mental repetition. Always use the same mantra; the mind will attune itself to the sound and rhythm and will focus more easily. A mantra is a powerful tool, channelling two aspects of the mind – the desires to see and to hear – which can interrupt the flow of concentration when not properly directed. As you repeat the sound, you listen to it and at the same time visualize its form.

You can also repeat a mantra and visualize any symbol of an uplifting nature. The symbol can be abstract or concrete. You can focus on light, the sun, or the sky, or on a symbol connected to your religious belief if you have one, such as Christ, Krishna, or Buddha; or the Star of David, the Cross, or OM. You can also focus on a positive quality like love or compassion, relating to it, not as an abstract concept, but as a living entity that you want to manifest through your actions and words.

Make sure that the object of your concentration is of an uplifting nature: it should have the inherent power to take your mind to the infinite. In the *Yoga Sutras*, Patanjali expands this idea even further by advising us to focus on anything of an agreeable nature, allowing unlimited scope for choice.

9 GIVING SPACE TO THE MIND

Allow the mind to wander at first – it will jump around, but will eventually settle into concentration, along with the concentration of prana. Initially, in your eagerness to control the mind, you may

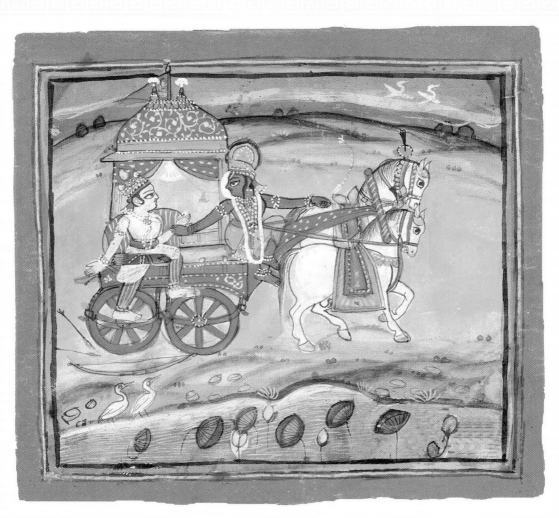

THE BHAGAVAD GITA

The *Bhagavad Gita*, or the Song of God, is one of the world's great books of wisdom, equal in depth and scope to such scriptures as the Bible and the Koran. Part of the great Sanskrit epic the *Mahabharata*, and consisting of eighteen chapters of 701 verses, it relates the dialogue between Lord Krishna and the warrior Arjuna, Krishna's greatest devotee (seen above). It symbolizes the eternal struggle between the downward pull of the instinctive, lower mind and the outward expansion of the spiritual essence in every human being. Its timeless wisdom is subtle and profound and as relevant now as it was when first written hundreds of years ago, offering a practical guide to a fulfilled life in today's fast-moving world. As a wonderful exposition of three of the main paths of yoga – *karma yoga* (the yoga of action), *bhakti yoga* (the yoga of devotion), and *jnana yoga* (the yoga of knowledge), it delivers a powerful message of hope, encouragement, and inspiration and is an essential companion to those seeking respite from the difficulties of everyday life.

be too forceful with it. If you focus too hard, a headache may develop. Relax deeply into the breath and focus more gently. We are often unaware even of our most obvious psychological habits and the power that they have over us. Be patient. There is a natural tendency to want a quick fix, but there is no easy way to bring the mind to a permanent state of silence and contentment. It needs to be freed very gradually from its many layers of emotional agitation. If the release is too sudden, there is a danger of being overwhelmed by the resulting reaction and you may decide to abandon the practice. Change has to happen consciously, progressively, and steadily to have a lasting effect.

So give yourself space. Be both firm and gentle with the mind at the same time. Educating your mind is similar to educating a child. Both love and strength are necessary. Arm yourself with patience. Develop a healthy relationship with yourself, avoiding both overindulgence and harshness. Realize that what you are attempting to accomplish is not easy and feel a healthy pride when you make a step forward, however small it may seem. As the *Bhagavad Gita* says, become your own best friend and feel compassion for that part of you which is struggling to regain a sense of wholeness.

As you give space to your mind, keep it under close observation, like walking a dog with an extended leash – the dog retains a sense of independence, but is quickly reminded that its freedom is limited when it wants to wander off. During the first few minutes of your practice, develop a relationship of trust with your mind by being patient and compassionate. Then you will find that the part of your mind that resists being told what to do will cooperate more readily.

10 DISASSOCIATING FROM THE MIND

If the mind persists in wandering, simply disassociate from it, and watch it objectively, as though you were watching a film. Sometimes the mind is resistant and continues living in its world of imagination. To start with, you may find this a little frustrating, even discouraging. If this is the case, try another approach suggested by Swami

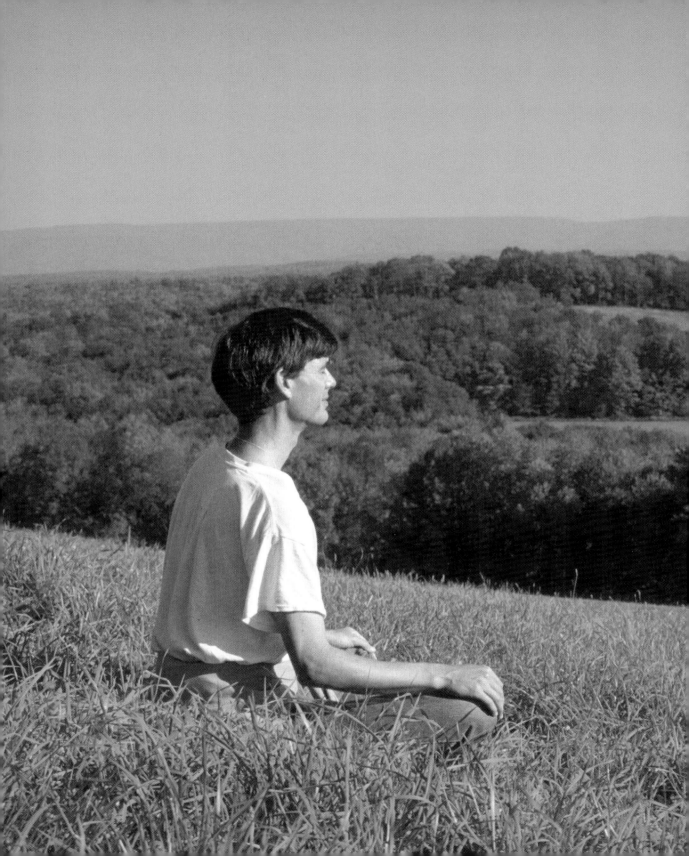

Sivananda – the attitude of non-cooperation. Watch your mind with the feeling: *I am not the mind, I am only the spectator of my mind.* If you find you are caught up in your own emotions and cannot let go, this practice of detachment or of witnessing will help. If you can sustain this mode of thought even for a few minutes, your mind gradually slows down. You stop feeding your emotions and thoughts with your consciousness and, since consciousness gives life to everything, the emotions and thoughts will simply have no energy to live, and will lose strength and intensity. Powerful discrimination and a good level of emotional strength are required to maintain a distance from your thoughts even for a relatively short time and may prove demanding for a beginner. However, try to practise a little each day, and a powerful new habit will gradually develop.

11 PURE THOUGHT

Sustained concentration leads into meditation. This occurs after many months and, in most instances, after many years of practice. The experience of meditation is explored in Section II of this book.

12 SAMADHI

Sustained meditation leads into *samadhi*, a state we enter when we have trained the mind to find absorption in consciousness itself. Samadhi is the highest state of meditation and the eighth step in the raja yoga system. Here, duality disappears and you enter the superconscious state. See Section II.

The stillness and calm of nature acts as a perfect setting for the practice of meditation.

CHAPTER TWO

THE YOGIC LIFESTYLE

By now you will have realized that meditation is not just a question of sitting cross-legged with your eyes closed. It is the ultimate goal of all yogic practices, and for full benefits it requires careful preparation both just before you start your practice and in your lifestyle as a whole. Adopting a lifestyle that will support your efforts to bring the mind within is not an easy task, and demands willpower and commitment of the heart, but the more care and attention you put into preparing yourself, the greater your success in meditation will be.

UNDERSTANDING THE GUNAS

In order to understand what this preparation requires, you need to be familiar with the yogic concept of the three *gunas*. The gunas are the three prime qualities of nature, which manifest in various combinations in all things. They are *sattva*, the quality of balance, purity, and harmony; *rajas*, the quality of action, passion, and dispersion of energy; and *tamas*, the quality of darkness, dullness, and inertia. These qualities are found everywhere in nature. They also manifest in your body, mind, and personality in general. This model of the three gunas is very useful in evaluating any situation or inner state and will enable you to understand why you find it difficult to focus and what you can do to remedy the situation.

In the state of sattva, the mind is able to focus within and is calm and clear. The body feels light. There is an inner sense of contentment and goodwill towards all beings. When the energy of rajas predominates, the mind is restless and scattered and the emotions are easily upset. The body will also manifest this restlessness and you feel uneasy and agitated, seeking relaxation and relief through the enjoyment of external objects. When tamas predominates, the energy is stagnant, the mind dull, passive, and indifferent.

Effort needs to be applied to increase sattva in all the aspects of your personality and your life, because only in a sattvic state of mind will you have the motivation and energy necessary to expand your consciousness and resist the negativities of the mind.

Ideally, your whole lifestyle should support your meditation practice. Meditation becomes a way of life. Everything you do, say, or think can be a help or a hindrance to your meditation practice. Every sattvic action, word, or thought will uplift your energies and bring you closer to the meditative state. Actions and thoughts of a rajasic nature will create agitation, passion, and greed and distract you from your goal. Actions and thoughts of a tamasic nature will dull and veil your mind, breeding carelessness and lethargy, destroying your motivation to uplift yourself. To experience the joy of expanded consciousness, you need to live your daily life with awareness.

DAILY EXERCISE

It is important to take good care of your body. Take regular exercise to keep it strong, flexible, and free from tension. Remind yourself that you need to be in good health to maintain the perfect stillness required for the practice of meditation. If your joints are stiff, if your muscles are tense and weak, if you suffer from illness and disease, you will find it difficult to keep your body quiet. If you are unwell, avoid drugs and medicines as much as possible, substituting natural cures when you can, but don't take this to extremes by refusing to take medicine if you really need it. It is much better to take medication for a few days than allow a problem to take hold. Remember that, even if you are ill, seriously or otherwise, you can still practise light meditation. The practice of meditation is the best medicine for any disease, as it energizes and purifies every cell and tissue in the body.

Half an hour a day of regular exercise such as brisk walking, swimming, cycling, or light jogging will keep the body robust, and half an hour – or, if possible, an hour – of *asanas* (yoga postures) will keep you supple, strong, and energized.

The practice of asanas is the best preparation for meditation.
The classical treatises on *hatha yoga* (the practice of asanas) state
clearly that the purpose of performing the many dozens of different
asanas is to prepare you to hold the meditative pose with ease for
an extended period of time. The benefits of practising the asanas on
the health of both body and mind are numerous and include
increased strength, flexibility, stimulation of the internal organs and
glands, and rejuvenation of the nervous system. In the astral body
there is an improved flow of energy and purification of the energy
channels. On the mental level there is an increase in concentration,
emotional balance, contentment, calmness, and a sense of
groundedness. On a deeper level still, the asanas expand our
consciousness and awareness of our connection to the universe.
Swami Vishnu-devananda recommends practising the twelve basic
asanas, always in the same order. Your session should start with an
initial relaxation lying on your back (see page 42), then a series of
five or six rounds of sun salutations, then the twelve basic asanas,
finishing with final relaxation.

Another very important practice is pranayama. Because of the
interrelated nature of the mind and the breath, pranayama is an
excellent preparation for meditation. As you make your breath
rhythmic and deep, the subtle waves of prana of which your
thoughts are made calm down. Pranayama purifies and energizes
the whole body, cleansing the respiratory system and stimulating
circulation. It massages the internal organs and improves their
functioning, relaxes the nervous system, and helps depression and
emotional imbalance. Pranayama also purifies the *nadis* or psychic
nerves, through which the prana flows, and this improved circulation
energizes the whole system and clarifies the mind.

We recommend that pranayama should be practised every day for
up to thirty minutes, either before or after your asana practice. The
basic pranayamas (see opposite) are *kapalabhati* (pumping breath)
and *anuloma viloma* (alternate-nostril breathing). An average daily
practice includes three rounds of kapalabhati and ten rounds of

PRANA AND PRANAYAMA

Prana is the universal principle of vital energy or life force found in all living forms and supplied by food, water, air, and sun. Its equivalent in Chinese philosophy is *chi*. In a human being, its first manifestation is the breath. The practice of pranayama (the fourth step of raja yoga) aims at increasing and controlling this life force. The mind is the internal manifestation of prana and by controlling the prana you can control the mind.

Anuloma viloma

Anuloma viloma is a powerful pranayama technique used to purify the nadis (see page 29) and to calm the mind. Air is rhythmically drawn in through the left nostril to a count of four seconds, retained by blocking off both nostrils for sixteen seconds, and exhaled through the right nostril for eight seconds. A full round is completed when air is then drawn in through the right nostril to the count of four seconds, retained for sixteen seconds and exhaled through the left nostril for eight seconds. The left hand rests on the left knee in chin mudra (see page 24) and the right hand is used to block off each nostril in turn; the thumb blocks the right nostril and the ring finger blocks the left. The first and middle fingers are tucked away into the palm of the hand. The eyes are closed and the mind is brought to focus on the point between the eyebrows. Start with two rounds, increasing to ten daily. You will experience a renewed vigour and a calmer, more balanced mind within a few days.

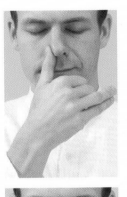

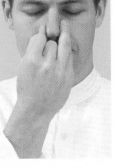

Kapalabhati

This is a powerful exercise that cleanses the respiratory system, invigorates the body, clears the mind, and improves concentration. Take two deep breaths through the nose. Then with each succeeding inhalation expand the abdomen and exhale rapidly, pulling in the abdomen. Repeat this in quick succession to establish a pumping action, with an emphasis only on the exhalation. A vacuum is created with the exhalation and the inhalation happens naturally, by itself. Do this pumping breath about thirty or forty times, then take two deep breaths and on the third breath retain the breath as long as you comfortably can (up to one minute). This constitutes one round. Three rounds on a daily basis will cleanse and strengthen the entire respiratory system increasing the intake of oxygen and thereby clearing the mind.

anuloma viloma. If you have time, you can also practise a few extra rounds of anuloma viloma in the evening before going to bed, to calm the nervous system and give you sound sleep. During the day keep up the practice of deep abdominal breathing, which will bring good amounts of prana into your system and particularly to your brain, helping you keep a calm and relaxed mind.

PREPARING BODY AND MIND

Getting up early to dedicate the precious time of early morning to meditation is a very important aspect of the practice. Your day should start on a positive note and meditation is the best way to do this. After a night's sleep, the body has accumulated tamas in the form of waste matter and a general sense of dullness. It is therefore important to cleanse it and to generate a new sense of sattva. The first step to achieving this is to bathe: a shower will not only give you a sense of physical cleanliness, but also an exhilarating sense of renewed energy and general freshness. Ayurveda (see right) recommends oiling the body afterwards, which will energize and protect it from outer energies. Your body should feel as clean and light as possible. If you meditate in the evening, try to shower before sitting for your practice. If this is not feasible, wash your hands, feet, and face. If you meditate immediately after a meal, you will find concentration difficult, as most of your energy goes to the digestive process.

The clothes you wear for meditation are also important and should always be clean, loose, and comfortable, and made of natural materials. Do not wear the clothes you use to meditate for other activities. The subtle energies generated by thoughts and emotions go into everything with which you are in contact. The clothes you wear during meditation will be charged with the vibration of the positive thoughts entertained in your practice. It is recommended to wear a meditation shawl made of cotton or wool. Your mind will associate wearing this shawl with the meditative state, increasing sattva. It will also prevent your energy from leaking out, keeping it

AYURVEDA

The ancient Indian healing system of ayurveda (literally translated as the science or knowledge of life) is considered to be the oldest medical system in the world. Ayurveda is closely allied to the practice of yoga and has been practised and refined for over 4,000 years. Recent research has shown that it formed the basis of the early Greek knowledge of physiology and medicine. Ayurveda is as relevant and effective today as it was in ancient times. It teaches us how to maintain and protect health, cure disease, and promote longevity. Based on balancing the physical, mental, emotional, and spiritual, it brings a renewed sense of harmony and wellbeing to anyone who follows its principles.

AGNI SARA

Agni sara is one of the six
kriyas (cleansing exercises)
and is particularly effective for
massaging the digestive system
and liver as well as toning and
strengthening the internal
organs. To do agni sara, take
a wide standing position, with
knees bent, hands pressing on
the thighs and looking down on
the abdomen. Exhaling deeply,
pull the abdomen in and up,
hold the breath, and rapidly
pump the abdomen in and out.
When you need to inhale, stop
pumping, take a normal breath,
exhale and continue. Three to
five rounds of ten to eighteen
pumpings are sufficient.

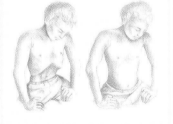

within your system. Wash the clothes you wear for meditation
regularly, keeping them separate and treating them with respect.

Because the mind is so easily influenced by the sensory impressions
it receives, it is important to feed it as much as possible with
positive and calming impressions before you sit to meditate. Avoid
sense stimulants of a tamasic or rajasic nature. To avoid stimulating
rajas, try not to talk before you meditate. This conscious choice of
not communicating with the outside world, called *mouna*, keeps the
energy introverted. Consciously rest your gaze on objects of a
positive nature such as a tree, natural scenery, or flowers for a few
moments. Or look at a picture of a divine being, a saint, or a sage.
Gazing at the steady flame of an oil lamp or a candle has a very
positive effect.

Your mental state is closely connected to the flow of energy within
your body. For this reason, it is advisable to practise a few minutes
of pranayama before you start. We recommend two to three
rounds of kapalabhati (see page 39) to clean the respiratory tracts
of excess mucus, stimulate the solar plexus, and improve the flow of
prana in the body, and a few rounds of anuloma viloma (see page
39) to balance your energy. Holding the headstand (see page 44)
for a minute or two will bring plenty of fresh energy to your brain
and greatly help in concentrating your mind. The practice of *agni
sara* (see left) will also stimulate the prana in the solar plexus and
sharpen the sense of being awake. If you still feel heaviness in your
body, do a few sun salutations (see overleaf) to move the prana.

Before starting and at the end of each practice session, it is important to relax in the corpse position. This allows the body to rest and reinvigorate completely in a very short period of time.

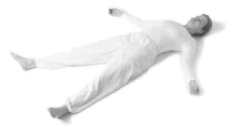

THE SUN SALUTE

The sun salute stretches and strengthens all the major muscle groups of the body. It improves the intake and flow of oxygen, stimulating the respiratory system and bringing increased blood flow, warmth, and energy to the whole body. The nerves are gently toned and allowed to relax, sense perception becomes more acute, and concentration is enhanced.

Positions 1 and 12 establish a state of concentration and calm;

Positions 2 and 11 stretch the abdominal and intestinal muscles, exercise the arms, and stretch the spine;

Positions 3 and 10 prevent and relieve stomach ailments, reduce abdominal fat, improve digestion and circulation, and make the spine supple;

Positions 4 and 9 tone the abdomen and the muscles of the thighs and legs and make the hips flexible;

Position 5 strengthens the muscles of the arms and shoulders;

Postion 6 strengthens the muscles of shoulders, arms, and chest;

Positions 7 strengthens the muscles of the upper back and arms;

Position 8 strengthens the nerves and muscles of the arms and legs and tones the spine.

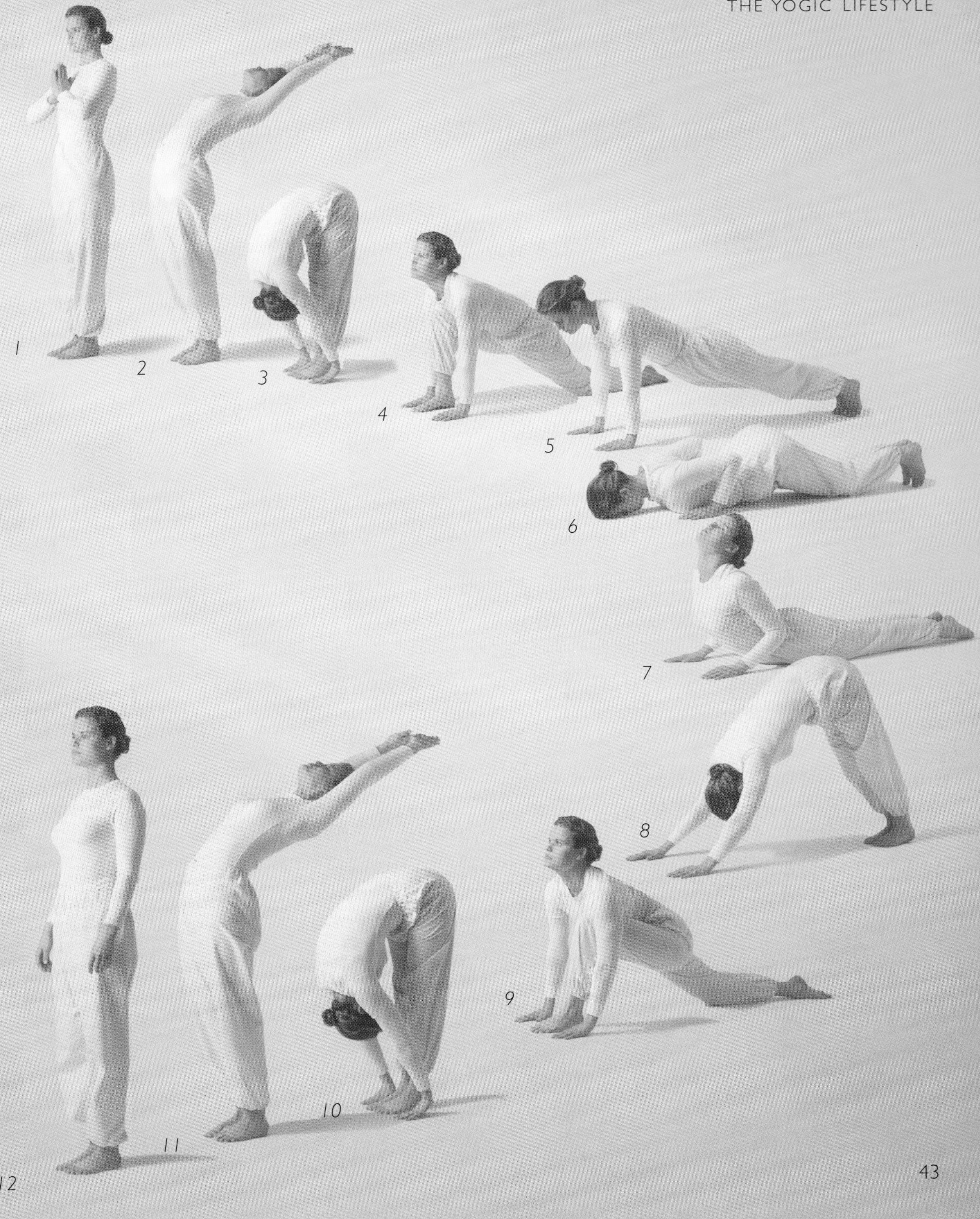

1

2

3

4

5

6

7

8

9

10

11

12

1 HEADSTAND

Strengthens the respiratory and circulatory systems

Improves disorders of the eyes, ears, nose, and throat; improves eyesight and hearing

Relieves varicose veins

Relieves kidney problems and constipation

Relieves pressure on the lumbar and sacral areas of the lower back

Encourages deep exhalation, removing toxins from the lungs

Increases hair growth through increased circulation to the scalp

Stimulates the pineal and pituitary glands, revitalizing the entire mind and body

Aligns the spine

Increases circulation to the brain, improving memory, concentration, and intellectual capacity

Counteracts nervous disorders and anxiety

Improves quality of sleep

Increases confidence

2 SHOULDER STAND

Prevents kidney disease, bone disease, and muscle weakness

Keeps the neck and spine strong and elastic

Relieves varicose veins

Massages the heart

Strengthens the throat and thoracic regions

Removes mental sluggishness

Cures insomnia and depression

Improves quality of sleep

Helps painful menstruation and gynaecological disorders

Purifies the blood and improves circulation

Regulates the thyroid gland in the throat. The thyroid regulates:
Metabolism and heat production
Protein synthesis
Growth and development
Heart rate and blood pressure
Calcium levels in blood and tissues

3 PLOUGH

Stretches the spinal muscles and ligaments and opens up the spinal discs, rejuvenating the entire spine

Nourishes the spinal nerves

Relieves and prevents back and neck arthritis and stiffness

Releases tension from the cervical region of the spine

Strengthens the muscles of the back, shoulders, and arms

Massages the internal organs

Relieves indigestion and constipation

Stimulates the liver and spleen

Reduces obesity

Relieves insomnia

Relieves constipation and indigestion

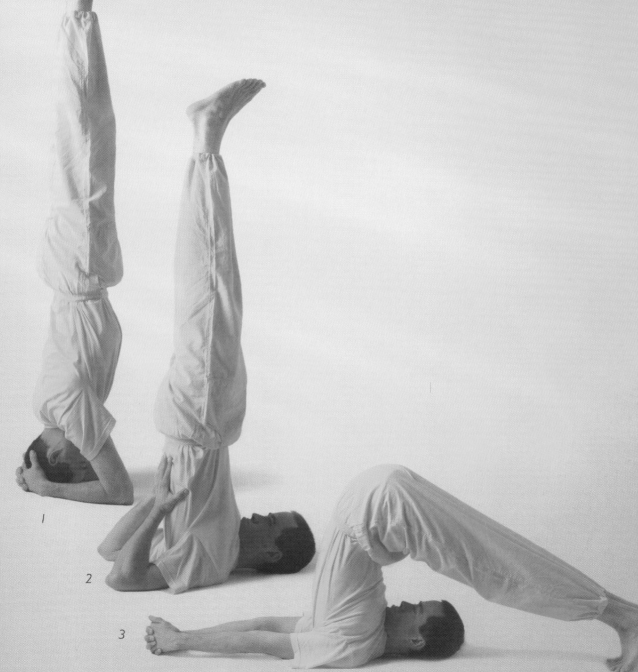

1

2

3

4 FISH

Removes stiffness from the cervical, thoracic, and lumbar regions of the back, bringing increased blood supply to these parts

Massages the neck and shoulders

Corrects round shoulders

Increases lung capacity

Relieves asthma

Stimulates and massages the parathyroid glands in the back of the neck, which helps prevent tooth decay and increases bone strength and plasticity

Stimulates and tones the pituitary and pineal glands

Regulates moods and calms the emotions

Relieves asthma

Strengthens and cleanses the respiratory system

Keeps the spine supple

5 SITTING FORWARD BEND

Reduces excess weight in the waist area

Reduces enlargement of the liver and spleen

Massages, stimulates, and tones the digestive organs, increasing digestive power

Massages the kidneys, liver, and pancreas

Regulates the functions of the pancreas, which controls carbohydrate metabolism and blood sugar levels

Regulates the intestines and increases peristalsis

Invigorates the entire nervous system

Stretches all the muscles in the back of the body

Increases flexibility in the hip joints

Alleviates disorders of the urino-genital system

6 COBRA

Increases flexibility of the spine, relieving curvature of the spine

Relieves asthma and other respiratory problems

Tones and massages the deep and superficial muscles of the back

Invigorates the nerves and muscles of the spine

Relieves lumbago and lower back pain

Tones the abdominal viscera

Tones the ovaries and uterus in women, relieving menstrual problems

Tones the adrenal glands

Relieves constipation

Relieves backache caused by overwork or long hours of standing

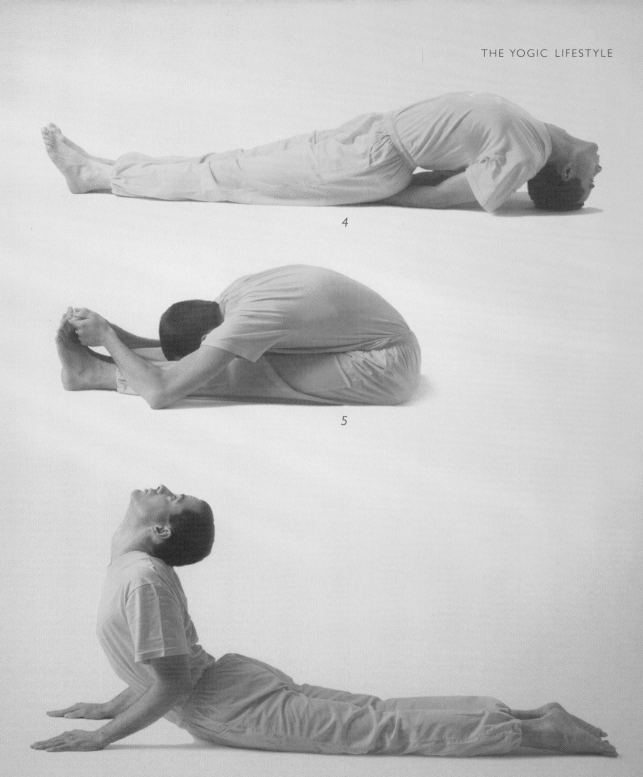

4

5

6

7 LOCUST

Relieves sluggish digestion

Strengthens the abdominal walls

Massages the pancreas, liver, and kidneys

Increases the blood supply to the neck and throat

Increases flexibility in the cervical region of the back

Strengthens the muscles of the upper back

Relieves lower back pain and sciatica

Stimulates digestion

8 BOW

Increases flexibility of the entire spine

Invigorates and massages the digestive organs

Removes abdominal fat

Relieves constipation, dyspepsia, and gastro-intestinal disorders

Regulates the pancreas, aiding those suffering from diabetes

Strengthens the abdominal muscles

Strengthens the respiratory system and relieves asthma

Prevents rheumatism of the legs, knee joints, and hands

Massages the back muscles

Keeps the spine elastic

Improves blood circulation

9 HALF SPINAL TWIST

Rotates the spine, keeping it elastic

Relieves lumbago and rheumatism of the back and hips

Tones and stimulates the sympathetic nervous system

Increases circulation

Stimulates the liver and the large intestine

Tones the gall bladder, spleen, and kidneys

Massages the digestive organs

Relieves constipation and indigestion

Regulates the secretion of adrenalin and bile

Relieves asthma

Strengthens the deep muscles of the back

Corrects stooping shoulders, bent back, and poor posture

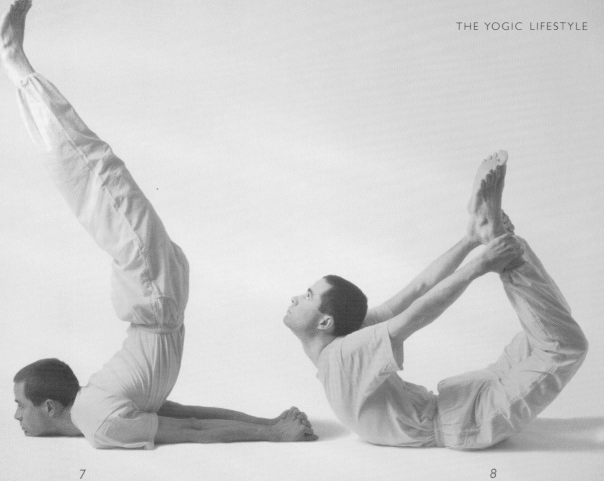

7

8

9

10 CROW

Strengthens the arms, wrists, and shoulders

Increases breathing capacity

Stretches the fingers, wrists, and forearms

Increases the powers of concentration

Removes sluggishness

Promotes mental and physical balance

11 STANDING FORWARD BEND

Increases the length of the spine

Mobilizes the joints, making the spine elastic

Invigorates the entire nervous system

Stretches the hamstrings

Increases blood supply to the brain

Removes excess weight from the waist

Makes the body feel light

Relieves constipation

Tones the spinal nerves

Relieves sciatica and low back pain

12 TRIANGLE

Tones the spinal nerves and abdominal organs

Increases peristalsis of the digestive tract

Promotes hip flexibility

Relieves nervous depression

Stimulates the appetite

Strengthens the pelvic area

Reduces excess weight from the waist

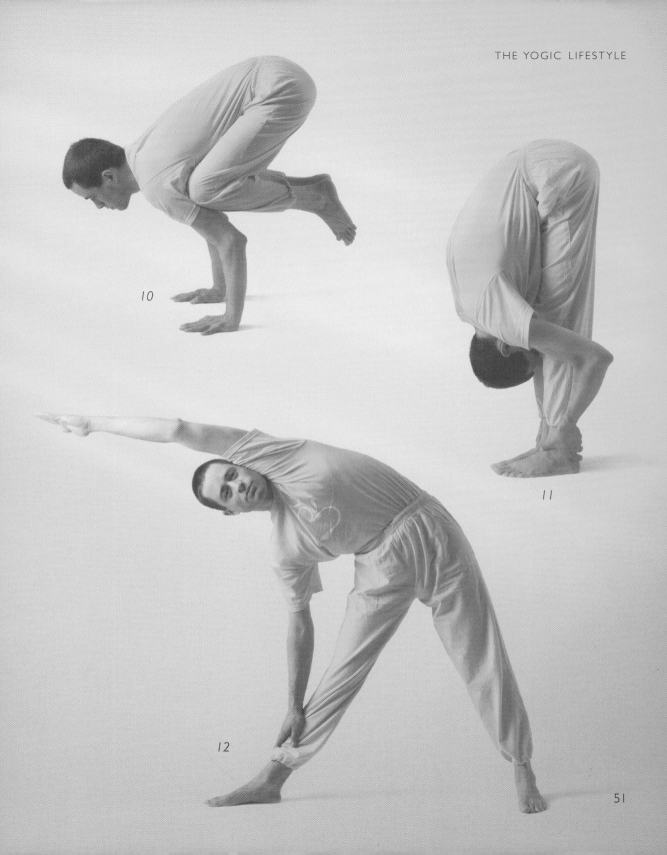

10

11

12

A PEACEFUL DIET

A poor diet can act as a severe hindrance to the practice of meditation. To have a calm and concentrated mind, we need to follow a sattvic diet. All foods have distinct energies that are used to build the human organism. Yogic science (like Western science) recognizes that the physical body is formed from food, but yoga goes one step further and states that the mind is formed from the subtle energies of food. What is consumed by the human body correlates directly to the efficiency with which the brain functions. Accordingly, if you eat food that is overprocessed, the mind will reflect the impurities in the food by becoming unbalanced. For example, studies show that certain red food colouring creates hyperactivity in children and that refined sugar can cause emotional

DIET AND AYURVEDA

We are bombarded from all directions with information and tips on nutrition and diet. Quite often we are unable to see the whole picture and are confused by the seemingly contradictory advice offered. Yoga can help the individual find a way through this maze. It advocates a pure vegetarian diet based on the ancient knowledge of ayurveda (see page 40). According to ayurveda, one of the foundations for good health is nutrition in harmony with our constitution, teaching us how important diet is in the treatment of diseases. Longevity, strength, energy, growth, complexion, and lustre all depend on a good digestive system and a good diet.

Ayurvedic hints on an ideal diet
It should taste good
It should satisfy
It should fortify the body
It should give both instant and lasting energy
It should be taken in proper quantity
It should boost vitality and memory
It should promote longevity.

Guidelines for healthy eating
Eat, seated, in a pleasant environment
Eat only after the previous meal has been digested (five to six hours)
Eat calmly and chew well
Drink a little hot water or herb tea with the meal
Avoid cold or iced drinks at all times

Be happy and cheerful when cooking and eating – your mood affects your digestive system and the energy of the food
Take meals regularly and at the same time daily. Avoid snacks between meals
Eat only about the equivalent of two handfuls of food. Fill the stomach half full with food, a quarter with water and leave a quarter empty for the expansion of gases
Avoid fruit and fruit juice with your meal
Do not eat late at night
Use food as medicine. You are what you eat
Give thanks for your food.

FASTING

Fasting is one of nature's greatest curative agents. It allows the system to rid itself of the toxins that build up in the body from pollution or unhealthy eating habits. Many people feel intimidated by the idea of fasting, fearing they will become weak and listless. On the contrary, a day's fast increases vitality and clears the mind. Memory improves and the body feels light and energetic. Overeating is one of the modern world's greatest problems and fasting allows the digestive organs, the stomach, liver, pancreas, and gall bladder a well-earned rest. In addition, fasting develops willpower and increases the power of endurance. Yoga recommends common sense if you do decide to fast. Drink plenty of water and herbal tea. If you feel full of toxins, take a rest while you fast, as detoxing can give you a headache and make you tired and irritable; otherwise, carry on with your life as normal. One day's fast a week or every two weeks is quite sufficient, and you should not fast for more than three days without medical supervision.

instability. These are just two of many hundreds of examples of substances that are often heedlessly consumed with no awareness of their effect on the body and mind. A person who meditates regularly must be particularly aware of these substances, as even on a day-to-day basis, diet affects the quality of meditation.

The optimum diet for a meditator is a simple one. This is not to say that meals should be unappetising, but there should be an absence of foods that negatively affect the mind. Hot and pungent spices, garlic, onions, too much salt, coffee, black tea, and meat all agitate the mind, making control of thought difficult. Other foods dull the mind, inducing a state of sleepiness instead of concentration. These include all precooked and overripe foods, as well as alcohol, and, though not taken as food, marijuana and cigarettes. It is not expected that every person will immediately make a radical change in diet, nor would this be advisable, but those who are sincerely interested in meditation may begin, for example, by phasing out meat and cigarettes. The practice of asanas and pranayama will make this much easier. Many detrimental habits will fall away by themselves, simply due to the change of consciousness that occurs in meditation.

Consider adopting a vegetarian diet. Some twenty years ago a person who refrained from eating meat was viewed with a certain amount of curiosity, if not suspicion. Today it is quite a different story. Health food stores and vegetarian restaurants abound and there is a growing awareness that our health is directly affected by what we eat. Many diseases can be cured by a change in diet or a short period of fasting to detoxify the system. This is true not only of physical disorders, but of many mental problems as well.

Contrary to popular opinion, vegetarians get plenty of protein. It is meat-eaters who consume too much. Animal protein contains a high concentration of uric acid, a nitrogen compound similar to ammonia. It is not water-soluble and cannot be broken down by the liver and so, though a certain amount is eliminated, the greater

proportion is deposited in the joints, resulting in arthritis. Hardening of the arteries and heart disease are two of the most common illnesses in the West, where the greatest amount of meat is consumed. The culprit is too much cholesterol which, if taken in excess, cannot be totally eliminated from the body. It forms fatty deposits along the walls of the heart and arteries, which gradually thicken until they are clogged and inflexible. Some think that merely switching from butter to margarine will solve the problem, but in fact any oil that has been hydrogenated is harmful. The major source of cholesterol, however, is not buttered toast for breakfast but the hundreds of kilos of meat and meat fats that people consume each year.

Start by shopping and cooking with a greater degree of awareness. Buy whole grains, fresh fruit and vegetables, and avoid additives, processed foods, and canned goods wherever possible. Buy one or two good books on nutrition and a vegetarian diet and within a few months a great change will take place. Try to eat a little less. Many people eat far more than is necessary, mainly out of habit, or to satisfy the senses. Overeating is the cause of the great majority of diseases encountered in modern society. Meditation becomes impossible when the stomach is overloaded; drowsiness sets in and sleep follows. Be moderate in the amount you eat. Your mind and body will feel light, alert, and full of energy.

Of all the common diseases, the one that strikes fear into most hearts is cancer. Many substances have been found to cause cancer in animals, but studies seem to indicate that the amounts of these substances consumed in food by the average person are insufficient to be carcinogenic. However, it is the accumulation of these poisons over a period of years that causes cancer. Innumerable chemicals are fed to and injected into animals to increase their weight and the profit they yield. Nitrites, food colouring, artificial hormones, and even arsenic are among the chemicals added to animal flesh before it goes on the supermarket shelf. These, along with additives in other foods, collect in the body and are stored in the tissues.

Cancer occurs when normal body cells react to these excessive toxins by mutating into cells that reproduce uncontrollably.

There are other practical and spiritual reasons for not eating meat. Four times more grain or soya is needed to feed animals bred for human consumption than to feed a person directly. This raises a moral question regarding the sharing of the world's resources. The vegetarian diet is also less expensive and results in the most efficient utilization of available land. Plants are the original source of energy for all living beings, as they store the energy of the sun through photosynthesis. Vegetarians take their nourishment from this powerful and life-enhancing original source.

It is also worth noting that our digestive system is not one of a carnivore. Our teeth are suited to biting and crunching vegetables, not for tearing flesh – we must age, tenderize, and cook meat before we can eat it. The human liver is proportionally smaller than that of a meat-eating animal and is not built to filter animal poisons. The alimentary canal, which is short in carnivorous animals in order to speed these poisons through the body, is long in humans, as it is in all vegetarian animals.

For a yogi, though, the main consideration in not eating meat is the basic principle of *ahimsa*, or non-injury. *Thou shalt not kill*, as the Bible says. Animals have feelings and a consciousness, just as humans do. Mass breeding and slaughter is cruel and unnecessary. In India a cow is regarded with great respect for the service it renders to society. It tills the fields, provides milk and its by-products for nourishment, and its dung is used for fuel and in building houses. An Indian farmer would never think of cooking his cow for dinner.

There is no doubt that you are what you eat. A subtle part of what is consumed becomes our consciousness. Those who change to a vegetarian diet notice a corresponding change in consciousness. A certain grossness disappears and awareness becomes more refined; the mind is more easily controlled. Then, with time and practice, success in meditation is assured.

CHAPTER THREE

CONCENTRATION

*Concentration is holding the mind
to one form or object steadily for a long time.*

PATANJALI, YOGA SUTRAS, III-I

Meditation becomes possible only when you have developed the ability to concentrate. The practice of concentration strengthens the thought currents, clarifies ideas, and energizes the mind. Ideas that were once cloudy and hazy become clear and definite. What was difficult, complex, and confusing becomes easy to grasp. You are able to work more, with greater efficiency and rapidity. Concentration strengthens the willpower and brings serenity, energy, a penetrative insight, powerful speech, the power to influence others positively, cheerfulness, and a sweet voice. Your mind will obey you and carry out all your commands. Sustaining the practice of concentration in the long term can also prevent or minimize the problems of senility.

THE FIVE STATES OF MIND

To understand the process of concentration we need to look at how the mind's waves function. Yoga teaches us that there are five different states of the mind.

1 Mudha

In *mudha*, the tendency of the mind is to see and cause suffering. In this tamasic state we deny happiness, projecting our own misery on to anyone who enters our field of awareness. Our creative energies are blocked and we feel trapped for ever, forgetting the very possibility of a higher and more expanded existence.

2 Kshipta

The *kshipta* state is rajasic and characterized by scatteredness. We experience pleasure and pain with our activity directed towards the satisfaction of our desires. We think little of the outcome of our

The power of a concentrated mind can be likened to the mighty force of water dammed.

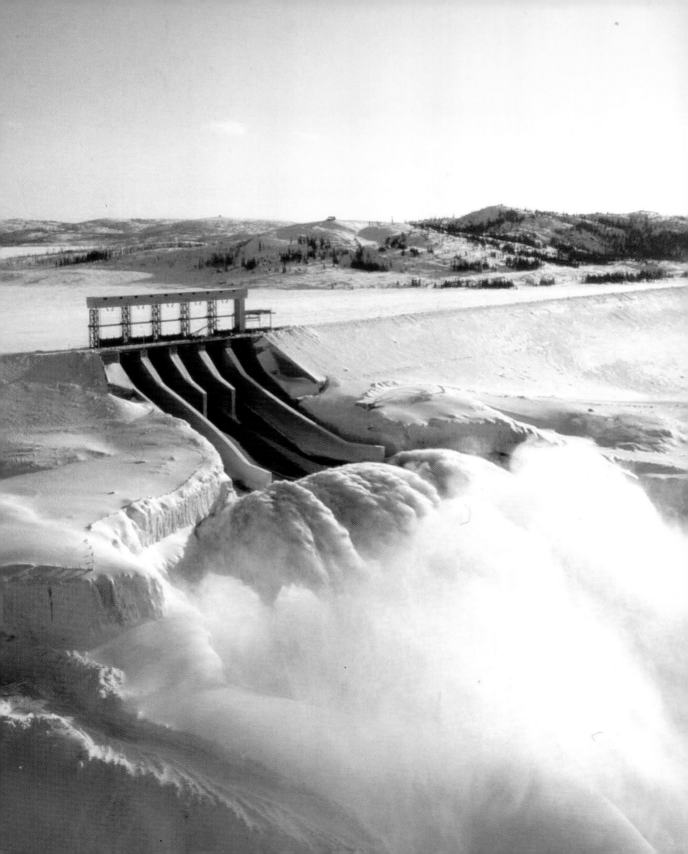

behaviour and even when warned about the probable negative consequences of an action, we find justification for it and do it anyway. We are fearful, greedy, selfish, and quite chaotic, running after pleasures and away from pain.

3 Vikshipta

In the *vikshipta* state, we struggle to draw ourselves inward. We make a conscious effort to gather the rays of the mind and focus them, sometimes successfully, sometimes not. We run again after pleasure and again we stop and return inward. This process of gathering the outward-going thought waves requires some effort, but success brings great satisfaction.

4 Ekagrata

In the *ekagrata* state, we reach one-pointedness of mind. There is no longer any need to struggle to gather our attention. We realize that there is more happiness in the state of concentration than in the experience of pleasure. Ekagrata is a sattvic state of mind.

5 Niruddha

In *niruddha*, which is also a sattvic state of mind, there is a suspension of mental activities and we experience supreme joy. This is what we experience in the state of deep meditation.

Our most familiar states are probably the depression of the mudha state, or kshipta, where our mind jumps to hasty and shallow conclusions and fails to gain a profound understanding of anything in life, including ourselves. The aim of concentration is to move from the states of mudha and kshipta to the one of vikshipta. We need to learn how to devote our entire mental energy to an object. The more concentrated the mind is, the more power is brought to bear on one point. The ability to attend fully to what we do is the key to success in any endeavour, and in meditation in particular.

This law applies universally: every force in nature moves more slowly and with less power when dispersed, than when it is

concentrated in one mass and directed through a single channel. When a river is dammed, its once-leisurely flowing water gushes out through the sluice with extraordinary force; when focused through a magnifying glass, the warm rays of the sun become hot enough to burn — such is the power generated by the concentration of force.

Everyone possesses the ability to concentrate to some degree, and each action makes demands on this ability, whether you read a book, write a letter, or wash the dishes. Some skills require quite a high degree of concentration. Operating on a patient requires the utmost attention from the surgeon. Deep absorption marks the state of the technician or architect engaged in drawing the minute details of a plan. There is also great concentration in force when playing a game such as chess. But today, due to fast technological development, poor diet, and other factors, the attention span of a great number of people, and particularly of children, has become very short. Problems such as poor memory and psychological disturbances are the result.

We need to understand how the mind operates in order to concentrate successfully. The first thing to note is that the mind has the power of attending to or perceiving only one thing at a time. However, because it moves from one object to another at incredible speed, we believe we grasp several things at once. If you listen to what someone says, you will not see that person at the same time. The mind connects to only one sense at a time and as a result we either hear or see, but not both simultaneously. The speed of the mind gives the impression that we are doing both.

If you are deeply engrossed in a book or a television programme, you hear no outside noises, not even your own name. If somebody approaches, you are not aware of it, nor do you smell the fragrance of the roses by your side. This is one-pointedness of mind or the ekagrata state. When you do try to do two or more things at the same time, you find that your work slows down. As the mental rays scatter, the energy dissipates.

Try to train your mind to give undivided attention to each situation in your life. Learn gradually to concentrate on the work at hand by shutting out all other thoughts and doing nothing haphazardly or in haste. When you eat, do not think of work; when you are at the office, do not think of home. The greatest impediment to attention is restlessness. When you start to practise, you will see your thoughts leap around in an uncontrolled way. Patiently and firmly fix the mind on one object alone. When it runs away, as it naturally will, pull it back gently again and again. With regular practice your ability to concentrate will deepen, you will accomplish tasks in half the time and with twice the accuracy, and you will experience great spiritual joy.

THE SENSES

We have already seen just how important a role our senses play in the practice of concentration. It is the senses that pull the mind outwards. There can be no success in meditation without training the senses to turn within. The senses are the avenues through which the mind's energy flows and in order to reduce the outward flow and its consequent waste of energy, their activity must be controlled. This control is known as *pratyahara*, the fifth step in the raja yoga system. Pratyahara works with the energy of the senses and is the foundation on which the practice of concentration is built. We are often unaware how strongly impressions from the senses influence our mind and mould our reactions and choices. In addition, Western culture has a powerful tendency to pull the senses outward, making the practice of pratyahara even more essential for those who want to develop spirituality in their lives.

Sense impressions are food for the mind. They determine the quality of our thoughts and actions. Watching violent films, for example, fills the mind with violent impressions that reflect in our consciousness and can turn into aggressive behaviour. The mind becomes toxic in the same manner as the body does when we feed it junk food. Negative impressions from certain television

programmes and films, from newspapers and magazines, and from rajasic or tamasic music are indigestible to the mind, making it dull and depressed. Consider reducing the number of newspapers and magazines you read and the amount of television you watch. Their effect is to stimulate the mind, increasing the desire to consume, and causing feelings of inadequacy. When the senses are filled with such negativity, the result is often disturbed sleep patterns, a craving for stimulants, and a lack of clarity, creative energy, and inspiration.

Pratyahara consists of withdrawing the mind from rajasic and tamasic impressions so that it is unaffected by them. It is a fast for the mind. Pratyahara also means filling the mind with positive sense impressions. Gazing at a flower, a tree, the sky, a flame, an image of God, or a spiritual symbol will create sattva in the mind. Try to expose yourself daily to such uplifting impressions. Use your discrimination during the day, and be selective about the kind of impressions you allow in. Consciously absorb positive impressions – the craving for rajasic sense stimulation will markedly diminish and your mind will clarify.

EXERCISES IN CONCENTRATION

Initially, train your mind to concentrate on external objects. Later on as you progress you will be able to concentrate on subtle objects like a chakra, an inner sound, or an abstract idea.

Below we offer some very effective exercises to help you develop your ability to concentrate.

Concentration on an apple

As a preliminary exercise in concentration, retire to a quiet room and sit in a comfortable cross-legged position. Close your eyes and visualize an apple. At first, there may be thoughts of its colour, shape, and size and its different parts such as the stem, skin, flesh and seeds. Through the law of association, ideas of other fruits may also enter the mind, for when the mind thinks of an object, it also thinks of its qualities and parts, which leads it further; when it thinks

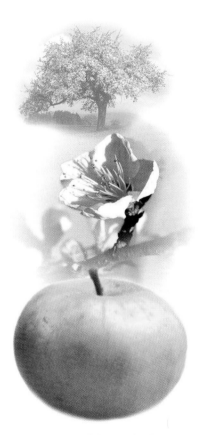

Think first of the apple, then its blossom, then its tree, expanding the point of focus but still keeping within the confines of your subject.

of a cause, it goes on to think of its effects. Soon, other ideas pop in and the mind begins to wander. It may think of meeting a friend at four p.m. It may think of shopping or the weekend's activities. It may go over an embarrassing incident from the previous day. Bring the mind back to the object in question gently but firmly. The aim of the exercise is to follow a definite line of thought, with no interruption, for a fixed amount of time. Start with one to two minutes and increase gradually to ten minutes.

Concentration on a flower

With your eyes closed, imagine a garden with many different flowers. Gradually, bring your attention to a single flower. Clearly visualize its colour, exploring and paying attention to its various qualities such as texture, shape, and scent. Hold the attention for as long as possible.

Concentration on a sound

Listen carefully to the ticking of a watch. Whenever the mind runs off, bring it back again and again to the sound. See how long the mind can be fixed continuously on the sound. Or listen to a group of sounds and select the most prominent one. Listen to it for some time, like a witness, without reacting to it. Then shift your attention to other sounds, one by one, for example from louder to quieter sounds and vice versa, becoming aware of the various qualities of each sound.

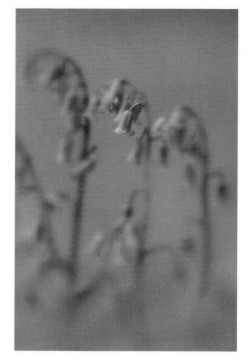

Out of a mist of bluebells, bring one flower sharply into focus and concentrate on its most delicate details.

Concentration on nature

During the day concentrate on the sky above. Lie down and gaze up into the sky. Feel the mind expanding while contemplating the vast expanse and you will feel a sense of elevation. At night concentrate on the moon or the stars. Or sit by the sea, and focus on the roaring of the waves, resounding like the sound of OM. Or concentrate by shifting your focus between objects near and far. For example, focus on a mountain, then on a tree, then on colours, and then on sounds.

Concentration on reading

Read two or three pages of a book with full attention. Test your concentration by stopping at the end of a page to see how much you remember of what you have read. Allow the mind to associate, classify, group or compare the facts of the subject matter – in this way you will acquire a wealth of knowledge on the subject. You will notice that when your mind is not focused, you will have difficulty assimilating the meaning and content of what you have read.

Concentration on an abstract quality

Relax the body and mind. Think about a quality like compassion. Feel its value, think how it can be expressed in everyday situations, especially under provocation. Follow a definite line of thought and recall the mind when it wanders. Think of great people who were the embodiment of compassion. Call upon this quality so it fills your heart, and from your heart let it flow out to the whole world, and think of yourself as perfectly compassionate.

Tratak on a candle flame

The yogic practice of *tratak* is an excellent exercise in developing concentration. It is one of six purificatory exercises in yoga called *kriyas* and concerns the sense of sight. It involves alternately gazing at an object or point without blinking, then closing the eyes and visualizing the object at the point between the eyebrows. Sit in a comfortable, steady cross-legged position. Place a candle at eye-level and arm's distance away. The room should be darkened and without draughts so that the candle flame remains steady. Relax your body and mind. Start by regulating the breath for two to three minutes. Then concentrate on the flame with open eyes for one minute. Blink as little as possible. After a minute or even less, tears may flow. Continue to look steadily at the flame without straining your eyes. Whenever the mind wanders, bring it back to the flame. Then close your eyes, relax the eye muscles and gently visualize the flame between the eyebrows, for an equivalent amount of time.

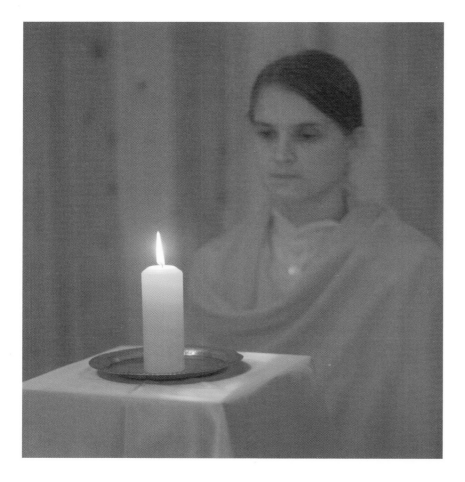

Tratak on a candle: visualize the flame at the point between the eyebrows, the ajna chakra, when you close your eyes.

Practise the exercise for only one minute on the first day, gradually increasing the length of time each week to up to half an hour. Be regular and systematic and, in time, you will be able to visualize the candle flame very clearly, even in its absence. This exercise stimulates the brain and the nerve centres, strengthens the eyesight, steadies the wandering mind and helps greatly in concentration.

Tratak on a picture

Sit in a comfortable position. Place in front of you an uplifting or inspiring picture or a spiritual symbol. Look at the image with a steady gaze. Then close your eyes and visualize it in the centre of

your heart or in the space between your eyebrows. When the picture fades in your mental vision, open your eyes and gaze at it again. Close your eyes after a few seconds and repeat the process.

Concentration on tasks

Strengthen your mind by focusing on tasks you do not like. By fixing your attention fully on a seemingly uninteresting object or situation, you start to see it in a new light and develop a liking for it. You realize that actually it is the state of sustained concentration itself that brings joy, not the object you are focusing upon. Your resistance will melt away and your mind become more open.

TIPS FOR DEVELOPING CONCENTRATION

Lessen the number of thoughts you entertain.

See the positive side of situations; a mind filled with negative thoughts will have difficulty concentrating.

Reduce excess: in physical or mental exertion, in talking, eating, or sleeping. Excess causes dullness and distraction and makes concentration difficult.

Whatever work you do, do it with full attention. Never leave work unfinished. Never do things haphazardly.

Never jump to hasty conclusions. Make sure you are fully focused before making decisions.

Learn how to relax.

Have an attitude of patience, cheerfulness, and tenacity. The practice of concentration demands willpower, untiring persistence, and regularity.

Do not give up the practice at any price. Success will eventually come. As Swami Sivananda says: "Nothing is impossible for a person who practises regular concentration."

CHAPTER FOUR

THE ART OF POSITIVE THINKING

Unless our mind is filled with positive thoughts, deep meditation is difficult to attain. When we harbour negative thoughts, our mind becomes agitated and restless, our actions disturbed and unbalanced. Thoughts of worry and fear are destructive to ourselves and to those around us. They poison the very source of life and destroy the harmony, efficiency, vitality, and vigour within us. Opposite thoughts of cheerfulness, joy, and courage heal and soothe. They improve our efficiency and increase our mental power. Yoga encourages us to live to our fullest capacity in accordance with the universal law of beauty and harmony. Such a life reflects an effort to share whatever we have with others and to actively promote peace and harmony in the world. In order to achieve this, we have to learn the most precious art of positive thinking.

When you ask most people what their goal in life is they will tell you it is to be happy, peaceful, and contented. This goal can take many forms, but in the Western world our tendency is to turn to external objects and events in the search for happiness. We think: *If I could have that car*, or *If I were just able to get that job*, or *If only I lived in the countryside*, or *If I could be with that person, then I would be happy*. We strive hard to acquire material possessions, a position with more status and responsibility, and an ideal home. And what happens when we attain our objectives? It is true we do experience momentary happiness. We feel at peace, the mind is still, there is a degree of satisfaction in our lives. But soon we tire of the new toy, it loses its attraction and the search for happiness begins again. Again we pursue another opportunity or object. Frequent change and acquisition is a way of life for many people, until, after many years of restlessness, we start to understand that external objects fail to bring the enduring happiness we seek. We grasp that the real source of happiness lies only within our own minds and that it comes from our approach and attitude towards the external world and not from the world itself.

Yoga teaches us that our thoughts are the real cause behind our success and happiness in life. The lives we live and the type of experiences we have are the direct result of the way we think. Whatever we are now and have achieved so far are the consequences of our thoughts. At first this may be too hard to accept, but as we explore the depths of our minds we discover it is true. As you think, so you become. Think that you are strong and you will become strong; think that you are weak and you will be weak. Good and evil, friend and enemy are only in the mind. We create a world of pleasure and pain out of our own imagination. These qualities do not proceed from objects themselves but belong to the attitude of the mind. One person's joy is another's sorrow.

Because thoughts are the source of all actions, they are the silent bricks that build our life. Thoughts mould our character and control our lives. Thoughts affect other people. We learn that we carry the responsibility for the quality of our thoughts, and that we can choose how to develop our thoughts and so choose the direction in which our life will go. We come to realize that we are the authors of our own lives. With our thoughts we hold in our hands the most powerful tools of transformation of our life. Thought is the most creative power in the universe and, when the potential contained in the power of thought is realized, it is the beginning of great spiritual growth in the individual.

In order to embark on the process of controlling our minds while engaged in our everyday activities, we need to understand the nature of thought and the laws under which it operates. We find that thought is subtle matter; it consists of a powerful energy, which, once created, has the ability to influence not just our own lives, but the lives of others too. A thought is like an object and, just like an object, has certain qualities. It has its own shape, weight, size, colour, texture, and power. We talk of a sharp mind, a blunt comment, a rounded personality, a broad vision, of feeling blue, light-hearted, or small-minded. Just as an apple can be given or taken back, so we can also give a thought to someone or take it back. We hear

ourselves say: *Give me an idea*, or *She's taken my idea*. Language abounds in such examples. These qualities of thought can be perceived by those who have developed a higher, psychic, yogic vision. For example, a spiritual thought is yellow in colour, whereas a thought charged with anger and hatred is dark red and shaped like a sharp arrow.

We also need to bear in mind the power of thought and the extent to which it can influence the world around us. A thought is not "just a thought", it is a living force. Swami Sivananda says a good positive thought is thrice blessed. Firstly it benefits the thinker, secondly it benefits the person about whom it is entertained, and lastly it benefits all of society by improving the general mental atmosphere. A negative thought, on the other hand, is thrice cursed. Firstly it harms the thinker, secondly it harms its object, and lastly it harms all of humanity by vitiating the whole mental atmosphere.

We live in a world of thoughts. We are surrounded by an ocean of thoughts and consciously or unconsciously draw certain thoughts towards us, at the same time sending out thoughts that are picked up by others. This is why people have experiences of ESP from time to time. Some wish to call these experiences coincidence, but they are not. The ability to communicate thought is developed to a higher degree, again in those who are said to be psychic, or who have great intuitive abilities. The mind has "drawing power". We attract towards ourselves, from both seen and unseen life forces, thoughts, influences, and conditions most akin to our own thoughts. We unceasingly attract to ourselves, knowingly or inadvertently, exactly and only what corresponds to our own dominant quality of thoughts. Like attracts like. If you think negative thoughts, these will attract negative thoughts from others. If you allow your mind to rest on good thoughts, you will attract good thoughts from others. Every person projects some kind of vibration. Some people are a pleasure to be with. They seem to have a certain energy that they share with others. Then there are those who are negative and depressed, who seem to actually drain the energy out of others.

Knowledge of how our patterns of thought develop is essential in order to gain control of the mind and to develop a more positive view of life. Yoga says that in a sense, the mind is like a CD. It contains grooves or impressions, which in Sanskrit are called *samskaras*. These samskaras form when certain thought waves, or *vrittis*, become habitual. For example, we pass a bakery and see a chocolate éclair in the window. The thought arises in our mind: *How delicious; I will buy that éclair.* If we ignore the thought and turn our mind to something else, no impression is formed, but if we identify with the thought, we give life to it. We buy the éclair and look forward to enjoying it as a treat that evening. Now, suppose we pass that same bakery every Tuesday and Thursday. Each time we go by we remember that wonderful éclair and buy another. This action, originally just a flash in the mind, has now become a force in our life and a samskara has been formed. Samskaras form when attention and attachment are given to a sensory impression. Samskaras are not necessarily negative. There can be grooves in the mind that are uplifting and others that bring you down. It is one of the purposes of meditation to eradicate destructive samskaras and to develop more positive ones.

We need to recognize that thoughts gain strength by repetition and that the stronger the thought the sooner it will be realized. If we constantly think we are, for example, fat, or shy, or not good enough, the samskara deepens and takes a strong hold on the mind. As we repeat the same thought, the samskara intensifies, and the actual power of the thought increases. As a result of this power the thought manifests in action. We find we start to eat more, we may refuse to socialize, we may not attempt to learn new things, we may become depressed. But if we think we are courageous, adaptable, modest, or considerate, we find that our actions will start to reflect these qualities. Our minds and hearts open and we discover the joy of living.

POSITIVE THINKING IN ACTION

How do we control a mind that, as Swami Sivananda says, is no better than a wild monkey, drunk, and stung by a scorpion? How do we stop the constant replay of past events, in which we rearrange them into a better drama, or the planning for an imaginary future? Why do we so often find ourselves caught in a situation with the same frustrations, the same problems? Having recognized how thought patterns develop, the next step is to become aware of the content of our patterns of thought; of what we are actually thinking. It is impossible to change, unless we recognize that change is necessary. We cannot lessen our anger unless and until we can see that we are angry. We perceive clearly what is happening in other people's minds and lives, but when it comes to our own, we show little insight. To develop this insight we need to witness or watch the mind (see Chapter One). One of the most effective ways of nurturing the ability to witness is to keep a spiritual diary (see Chapter Nine). The practice requires patience and perseverance, but gradually we watch ourselves in action, almost like a character in a film. We see when anger arises or when we worry, or when we avoid certain situations or people, allowing us the opportunity to change. Observing how other people act and then asking ourselves honestly if we conduct ourselves in the same way will also give us insight into our own behaviour.

Many methods are used in yoga to raise the vibration of our thoughts. These include asanas and pranayama, concentration techniques, the repetition of mantras, introspection, and self-analysis. One of the great techniques for strengthening positive thinking is the practice of thinking the opposite. We habituate the mind to contraries and learn to replace negative thoughts with positive ones. Hatred ceases not by hatred but by love. We examine our character and pick out a negative trait in it, and then think of its opposite. Let us say we suffer from irritability. The opposite of irritability is patience. We sit down every morning at a certain time in a meditative position for fifteen minutes and think of

patience. We think of its value and its practice under provocation, remembering one incident where patience was needed, then another, thinking as steadily as we can and bringing the mind back when it wanders. We think of ourselves as perfectly patient and end with a vow: *This patience which is my true being, I feel and will act on from today.* For a few days there may be no perceptible change. We are still irritable. But if we continue practising regularly every morning, soon, when irritation manifests, the thought will flash into the mind: *I should have been patient.* Still we continue the practice. After a while thoughts of patience will occasionally arise when irritability appears and the outer manifestation will be checked. Still we continue the practice. The irritable impulse will eventually weaken and patience will become our normal approach towards annoyances. We can use this powerful method to develop various virtues such as sympathy, self-restraint, purity, humility, benevolence, nobility, and generosity.

One of the great practices of all spiritual traditions to make the mind positive is to try and lessen desires. Desires by themselves are harmless, but they are strengthened by the power of imagination or thought. Desire generally begets desire in an endless cycle that creates restlessness and greed in the mind. An unsatisfied desire causes frustration and anger and can lead to disharmony and enmity. Should a desire manifest in the mind and be recognized as unproductive, practise bringing the attention of the mind to something else so that the samskara does not develop. Desire is a state of want. All desires spring from the desire to be loved. As long as we feel empty within, there will always be a desire to fill this emptiness with something from outside: material objects, food, relationships. We need to change our focus and connect again with the source of love within our spiritual heart.

Visualization and affirmations are powerful methods of changing thought patterns. Suppose you want to develop courage. When driving, walking, washing-up or waiting for the bus, assert mentally: *I am courageous, I have a strong will*, for ten minutes with deep

concentration. Keep notes in your pocket reminding yourself that you are courageous. Visualize yourself being courageous just before you face a situation about which you are anxious. You will see the fear melt away. When confronted with the difficulties of everyday life, see them as challenges, not obstacles. You do not have to look on failures negatively. A baby falls a thousand times before learning to walk. He does not give up until he achieves his mission. Similarly, we can see each failure as a stepping stone to success, as one step nearer to our goal. We can face situations with fortitude and courage. Swami Sivananda says: "The soul attracts that which it secretly harbours and also that which it fears." Until we confront our fears, they will pursue us. They may take different forms, but the essence of the fear will remain the same. Practising courage will allow us to face the fear. How often are we taken by surprise by a situation about which we have worried, only to find that we handled the occasion with much more skill and fortitude than we thought we had? The imagination plays havoc with our minds, creating worry and anxiety and preventing us from living in the present. Many of us feel that our lives are half-lived, that we live "on the periphery". The moment we stop thoughts of the future and the past and put our full attention on the present, we find an enriching and rewarding life lying in wait.

Positive thinking is not just a desirable spiritual practice but a necessity. Swami Sivananda urges us to strive ceaselessly to eradicate negative thoughts and develop positive ones. Without positive thinking peace in the world is not possible. We can think positively only if we have a higher vision, living in the awareness of the oneness of all of creation and understanding that life is to be lived in an ethical, selfless, and giving way. Unless we are able to put the tenets of such thinking into practice, there cannot be tangible changes made in our own life, or in the world. The benefits of our positive thinking will radiate to everyone as we all share the same world of thoughts. Once we master the art of positive thinking, we are happy, harmonious, and peaceful and a powerful meditation practice will follow.

When evil thoughts arise,
such as injury or falsehood,
whether they are done, caused to be done,
or approved of through
greed, anger, or delusion;
whether they are of slight, medium, or
great intensity and in infinite ignorance
and misery, take to the method
of thinking contrary good thoughts,
or habituate the mind to contraries.

PATANJALI, YOGA SUTRAS II-34

CHAPTER FIVE

MANTRAS, WORDS OF POWER

Meditation happens only when our minds are able to focus fully on a single object, and this is possible only when the mind is filled with sattva. If tamas prevails, the mind is dull, and when rajas dominates, the mind is restlessly chasing pleasure. A sattvic lifestyle will help to eliminate some of the qualities of tamas and rajas that predominate in an untrained mind. But we also need to work with the mind directly. One of the most powerful and efficient tools used in the yoga tradition to achieve this is a *mantra*. A mantra is a sacred word charged with spiritual energy. The word *mantra* is made up of two Sanskrit roots: *man* means to think and *tra* means to protect or to release from the bondage of the phenomenal world, or from negative thought patterns.

The science of mantra is very complex. In the modern world the power of sound is just beginning to be used in physical therapy and its potential is being tapped in other fields. However, Indian sages had this knowledge many thousands of years ago. They used sound in its gross and subtle states to penetrate the planes of human consciousness and cure diseases, remove obstacles, and reach the vibration that is the supreme experience. The power of mantra repetition reinforces the spiritual seeker's determination and ability to do spiritual practices. It develops detachment and wisdom in life, removing anger and greed and other failings that obscure our innate purity. Just as a mirror can reflect only when clean, the mind can reflect higher spiritual truth only when negative thoughts have been removed. Even a small amount of recitation with feeling and one-pointed concentration on the meaning of a mantra destroys negativities. Revealing the supreme essence to the meditator's consciousness, it confers illumination and supreme joy.

WHERE DO MANTRAS COME FROM?

According to modern-day physics our universe began with the Big Bang, a sound emanating from the void, whose vibrations have

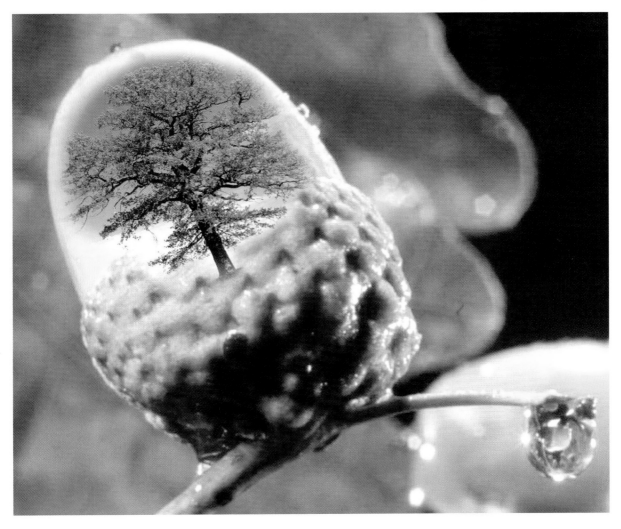

The oak tree lies dormant within the acorn – latent energy contains the potential of all form.

slowly evolved into the form of the universe as experienced today. The Christian tradition agrees with scientists that the universe was created by sound – "In the beginning was the Word, the Word was God and the Word was with God." In yogic cosmology and the writings of yoga the Big Bang is called the *Sabdabrahman*, the Sound of God. Yoga states that before the creation of the universe, there exists latent energy known as *shakti*, containing the potential of all form. Just as the oak tree lies dormant within the acorn, so the world of form lies within this shakti, awaiting manifestation. The first sound, the vibration of Sabdabrahman, is the energy that splits and

अ आ इ ई उ ऊ
ऋ ॠ ऌ ॡ
ए ऐ ओ औ अं अः
क ख ग घ ङ
च छ ज झ ञ
ट ठ ड ढ ण
त थ द ध न
प फ ब भ म
य र ल व
श ष स ह

The letters of the Sanskrit alphabet. For a key to transliteration, see page 151.

expands into wavelengths and eventually manifests as fifty articulate sounds or *varnas*. These combine and transform into the world of form, as all form is a manifestation of sound. These fifty primeval sounds, the foundation of all the forms of the physical world, have faded through time and are lost to memory. The Sanskrit language, however, is directly derived from them and of all languages it is the closest approximation to them. Sanskrit is also known as *devavani*, the language of the gods. Each mantra is made up of a combination of sounds derived from the fifty letters of the Sanskrit alphabet and is either a name of the Absolute, or an abstract formula.

Mantras have always existed in nature in a latent state, as sound energies, and cannot therefore be created or tailor-made for the individual. Just as gravity was discovered, but not invented, by Newton, mantras were revealed to the ancient masters in their deepest meditations when they tuned into higher levels of consciousness. The mantras have been codified and handed down from master to disciple through the ages. The yogic tradition is only one of many that has the Sacred Word as the core of its spiritual practice. Others include the traditions of the ancient Egyptians, the Buddhists, the Judaeo-Christians, the Sufis, and the Muslims.

HOW DO MANTRAS WORK?

How can the sounds of these mantras have such powerful effects on our consciousness? In order to answer this question, we need to look at the inherent power of sound. Sound has a definite and predictable effect on the human psyche and body. It can generate ideas, emotional reactions, and experiences. Merely by hearing words, we can feel pleasure or pain. If somebody shouts: "Fire! Fire!" we immediately tense, reacting with panic or freezing in fear. At the other end of the sound spectrum, we have all experienced the healing power of music. Listening to harmonious music can change our state of mind almost instantaneously. It opens the heart and soothes the soul. Sounds have other powers too. Their physical vibrations can produce predictable forms and various combinations of sounds produce complicated shapes. Experiments have shown that notes from certain instruments trace out precise geometrical figures on a bed of sand. In order to produce a particular form, a specific note must be generated at a particular pitch. Repetition of the exact note and pitch creates a duplication of the form. Sound is thus potential form, and form is sound made manifest. Everything in the universe vibrates on a specific wavelength and that wavelength can be manipulated. For example, when the pitch of the human voice is increased to a certain height, it can shatter glass.

Speech is our main means of communication with the world. The words we receive from others have a deep influence on our mental state. For instance, a negative statement heard again and again in childhood will create a negative conditioning that will remain with us in adulthood and will be difficult to break. A mantra has the power to release such emotional blockages, which are stored in the subconscious mind in the form of stagnant energies. The vibrations of the mantra release the blockages by resounding in our own subtle bodies because they are the sounds of our chakras. As you repeat the mantra, you stimulate the prana in the chakras, which releases energy from them. This in turn causes the mind to vibrate at the same level as the mantra, balancing and harmonizing the individual and uplifting the mind to higher levels of consciousness.

When repeated over a long period of time, the mantra creates a new energy pattern in the mind, eventually replacing the negative impression. Thus a mantra energizes the mind and helps us deal with our psychological problems and negative conditioning much more efficiently and directly than intellectual analysis can.

THEORY OF MANTRA REPETITION

The theory of the power of mantra repetition holds that by repeating the syllables with accuracy, and by attuning to the wavelength of the mantra, we are led from the gross plane of articulate sound back to the energy of the supreme consciousness or cosmic power. As cosmic power made manifest in sound, the vibrations produced by the tones of a mantra are important and pronunciation needs to be precise. If translated, a mantra ceases to be a mantra because the new sound vibrations created by the translation are no longer the vibrations or the body of the supreme consciousness and therefore cannot evoke it. The ancient sages were well aware of the inherent power contained in sound, and they knew that by tuning into these sounds they would be led to higher levels of consciousness. Repeated verbally or mentally, a mantra lifts one to a state where one does not just experience bliss, but becomes bliss. This is the true experience of meditation.

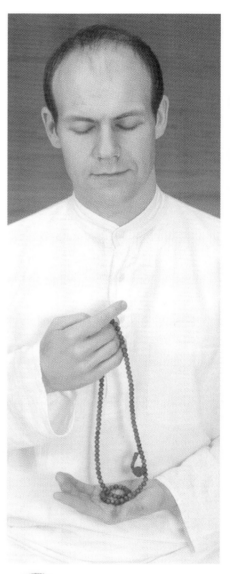

The mala is similar to a rosary and is used in japa, mantra repetition. The large bead is called the meru. When this is reached the mantra has been repeated 108 times and the mala is completed.

HOW TO USE A MANTRA

The practice of mantra repetition is known as *japa*. There are various practical aids to progress in japa that have been used for thousands of years and are based on sound psychological and natural principles. The rolling of rosary beads is the form of japa most familiar to the West. A *japa mala*, similar to a rosary, is often used in mantra repetition. It fosters alertness, acts as a focus for the physical energy, and is an aid to rhythmic, continuous recitation. It consists of 108 beads of the same size and an additional bead, the *meru*, which is slightly larger than the others. The meru bead signals that with one mantra recited for each bead, japa has been done 108 times and the mala has been completed. The fingers should not cross the meru. When you reach the meru, you reverse the beads in the hand, continuing to recite the mantra and moving the mala in the opposite direction. The thumb and third finger roll the beads; the index finger, which is psychically negative, is never used. The mala must not be allowed to hang below the navel and should be worn around the neck or wrapped in a clean cloth when not in use.

Start repeating the mantra with eyes closed and concentrating either on the *ajna chakra* between the eyebrows or on the *anahata chakra* of the heart. Try to pronounce it distinctly and without mistakes. Repetition must be neither too fast nor too slow and thought must be given to its meaning. It is best to synchronize the repetition with your breath. Increase your speed only when the mind begins to wander. As the mind will naturally tend to drift away after a time, or become tired, it may be necessary to introduce variety and so the mantra can be repeated aloud for a while, then whispered, and then recited mentally. Audible repetition, which is advantageous in shutting out distractions, is called *vaikhari japa*; whispering or humming is *upamsu japa*; and mental repetition, the most powerful form and requiring keener concentration, is called *manasika japa*. Even mechanical repetition that is devoid of feeling has a great purifying effect; feeling will come later, as the process continues.

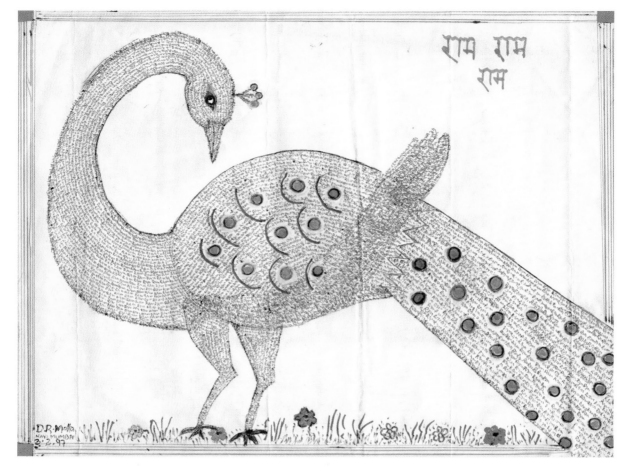

राम राम राम

In the beginning you may find it difficult to sustain the practice
for more than a few minutes. The mantra may sound meaningless,
mere syllables and nothing more. But if you persevere without
interruption, the mantra works itself into your consciousness and
you will start to feel the benefits within a few days. When you have
finished the practice, try not to immerse yourself immediately into
everyday activity. If possible, sit quietly for a few minutes, allowing
the vibrations to settle. As you get back into your daily routine, the
spiritual vibrations will remain intact. Try and maintain this current at
all times, no matter what you are doing. You can repeat your mantra
at work, while doing mundane tasks at home, or when caught in
traffic. You can use mental japa to take your mind away from

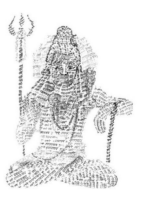

80

negative thoughts or from living in the past or future. Once you succeed in repeating the mantra throughout the day, a deep sense of peace will begin to permeate your consciousness.

Mantra writing, known as *likhita japa*, is another form of japa. Write your chosen mantra daily in a notebook dedicated to the purpose. Write it for ten to fifteen minutes, keeping complete silence and concentration. As you write, mentally repeat the mantra to intensify the impression in your consciousness. Likhita japa greatly helps to develop concentration and leads to meditation.

MANTRA INITIATION

Mantra repetition will be more efficient once you have been formally initiated into a mantra by your spiritual teacher (see Chapter Ten). Mantra initiation is the spark that ignites the dormant spiritual energy in every human heart. Once lit, the fire is fed by daily japa meditation. Only those who are pure can give initiation and it is important that you find a qualified teacher. For a teacher to successfully implant the mantra in your heart, he must have already broken its power. Breaking the power of a mantra means that one has meditated and obtained the mystic experience of the supreme essence through it, making its power one's own. At the time of initiation, the teacher arouses the mantra's *shakti*, or power, in his consciousness and transmits it, along with his own energy, to the student. If there is a psychic affinity between you and the teacher and you are receptive, you will receive the radiant mass of energy in your own heart and your practice will be vastly strengthened. Although it is customary for the teacher, when giving initiation, to accept voluntary offerings of fruit, flowers, or money, the selling of mantras is strictly against all spiritual rules.

CHOOSING A MANTRA

For those new to meditation the process of choosing a mantra can appear daunting. In fact it simply requires opening your mind to concepts that may be quite new and strange to you now, but will seem like old friends within a few months of practice.

A study in concentration and devotion. Here a peacock, symbol of Krishna and destroyer of the lower nature, is depicted with Vishnu's mantra Om Namo Narayanaya.

Lord Siva in likhita japa, lovingly drawn by repeating Lord Siva's mantra, Om Namah Sivaya.

You can select a mantra that feels appropriate yourself, but if you are not sure of your choice, your teacher will help you. If you are not able to go through initiation with a teacher (see above), daily mental repetition still has a strong purificatory effect, although it is not as powerful as after initiation. There are two types of mantras in which you can be initiated.

Saguna mantras

Saguna mantras invoke the name of a specific deity of the yogic tradition. Every true mantra fulfils certain conditions. Among them are that it should have a specific meter; it should have been revealed originally to a sage who achieved self-realization through it and handed it down to others; and it should contain a dynamic divine power within its sound structure. If you choose a saguna mantra, it helps to visualize the form of the deity that the mantra invokes as you repeat it, although you can also visualize the physical form of your teacher, or anything that is uplifting to you.

To understand the concept of a deity, it may be helpful to see him or her as one aspect of the one supreme essence, or energy, or consciousness. The grandeur of the Absolute is too vast for the mind to comprehend at the beginning of meditation practice, but the deity manifests it in a form that can be grasped. Each deity, complete within itself, represents an aspect of the whole. For example, Saraswati is the deity of wisdom, the arts, music, and literature. She represents that energy that undoubtedly exists in the world and manifests as an intellectual or artistic temperament. People of this temperament are drawn to that energy and may take her mantra for their meditation practice. If we compare the supreme essence to a mountain, each of the many paths to the top can be viewed as one aspect of this essence. The mountain itself is one mountain and the summit is the same. After reaching the top, you will have the vision of the totality. These different deities or aspects arise from the need for multiplicity in approach to the supreme essence. Various temperaments are attracted to different

manifestations of this essence. Each mantra has the same power in that it will lead you to the supreme essence; none of the mantras offered here is more powerful than any other mantra.

Nirguna mantras

People are of many different temperaments and not all are drawn to a personal deity. Some perceive the universe as diverse energy patterns, connected and interrelated, and stemming from a single source or primal cause. *Nirguna* mantras have no deity attached to them and appeal to those who are drawn to the abstract nature of supreme consciousness. We use nirguna mantras to assert identification with all of creation, a union with the unmanifest pure consciousness that underlies and permeates all existence. As with saguna mantras (above), to steady the mind further, visualization of an uplifting form will be of help during the repetition.

MANTRAS FOR JAPA

When choosing a mantra you will need to feel some kind of compatibility with it. You may like the sound, or the meter, or feel some affinity to the energy or deity that the mantra invokes. You need not worry that you will be choosing the "wrong" mantra; the one that you are instinctively drawn to, for whatever reason, will be right for you. Once chosen, your mantra should not be changed. It becomes your theme song and its vibrations become your own as it draws you closer to the supreme essence.

We offer here a selection of mantras that have been passed down from teacher to disciple over many thousands of years. We have given an explanation of each mantra as a guide to help you select one for your own practice. Please see the Key to Sanskrit Transliteration on page 151 for a guide to pronunciation.

SAGUNA MANTRAS

OM Sri Maha Ganapataye Namah

Prostrations to the Great Lord Ganesha

Ganesha is symbolized as the elephant-headed god who represents strength and fortitude, wisdom, and perfect control of the senses. He is the cosmic energy which, when invoked, can remove obstacles from our path and bestow success in our meditation. He also symbolizes all beginnings. His name is invoked before any activity is undertaken, so that it may be carried through with the right spirit and brought to successful completion.

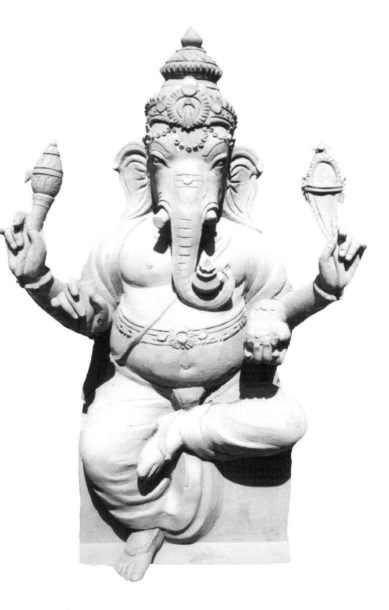

Om Śrī mahāgaṇapataye namaḥ

ॐ श्री महागणपतये नमः

OM Namah Sivaya

Prostrations to Lord Siva

Siva is the transformative energy of the universe. He is worshipped by those who have an ascetic temperament and are keen on remembering that everything is ever-changing. Siva is the Cosmic Dancer, whose energy breaks up the universe at the end of each age and brings it back to a non-manifested state. He represents the process of the old making way for the new. On a personal level, Siva's energy destroys our lower nature, making way for positive growth. Siva is the breaker of all limitations. He is also often represented as a yogi in deep meditation, unaffected by the world around Him. The snake that He wears around His neck as an ornament symbolizes the kundalini energy that is fully awakened in Him and over which He has perfect control. Siva is said to be very compassionate, ever ready to help those who tune into Him with respect. If you have reclusive tendencies and are determined to eradicate your negative qualities, or if you are drawn to abstract forms of thought and have a love of solitude and detachment, then you may be attracted to the Siva mantra.

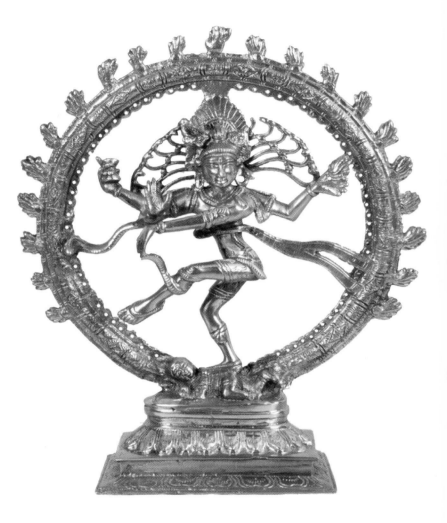

Om namaḥ Śivāya
ॐ नमः शिवाय

OM Namo Narayanaya

Prostrations to Lord Vishnu

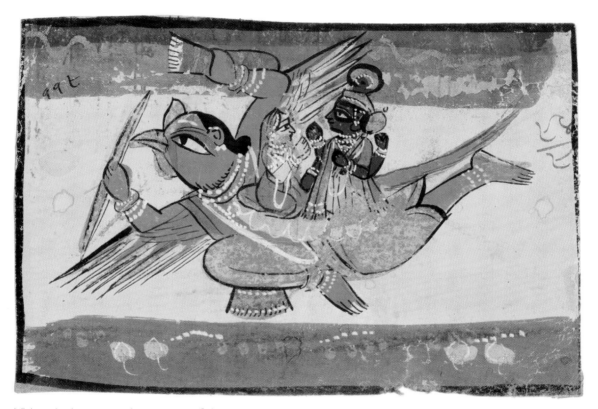

Vishnu is the preserving energy of the world. After the creation, it is the energy of Vishnu that maintains order in the universe. It is Vishnu who regularly takes on a human form and incarnates on earth to benefit humankind by reawakening in us the sense of *dharma* or righteousness. He symbolizes all goodness and compassion. People who are closely involved in the running of the world and in maintaining the harmony of life are drawn to this energy.

Om namo nārāyaṇāya
ॐ नमो नारायणाय

OM Namo Bhagavate Vasudevaya

Prostrations to Lord Vasudeva

This is the mantra of Lord Krishna. Lord Krishna is one of several incarnations of Vishnu. His multi-faceted personality draws spiritual seekers of varied temperaments. One part of His personality is pure playfulness and joy: many relate to Him as the mischievous child absorbed in divine play in the forests and fields of His birthplace, Vrindavan, bringing delight through His unpredictable and adventurous nature. Others see Him as the incarnation of divine love, ever engaged in teaching His devotees the art of perfect self-surrender. As such, He attracts devotional people who see the Absolute as infinite and all-loving and who are concerned with the welfare of others. Most people know Him as the inspired giver of the wisdom of the *Bhagavad Gita*, one of the greatest of all yogic scriptures. There He appears in His full glory. Through His dialogue with His devoted disciple, Arjuna, He teaches the world the art of equanimity and detachment in the midst of life's most challenging crises.

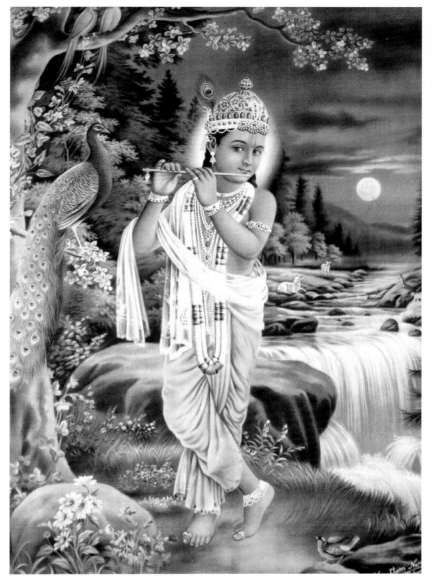

Om namo bhagavate vāsudevāya

ॐ नमो भगवते वासुदेवाय

OM Sri Ramaya Namah

Prostrations to Lord Rama

Rama, another incarnation of Vishnu, took life on earth for the purpose of upholding righteousness and rewarding virtue. The story of His life is the subject of the great epic the *Ramayana*. Rama lived a life full of perfection and responsibility and He and His wife Sita epitomize the ideal devotional relationship between husband and wife. Someone who is married and to whom family, responsibility, order, and ideals are vitally important may be drawn to Rama, who is the ideal son, husband, and lawgiver. Those with a strong sense of duty will feel drawn to His energy. As an incarnation of self-sacrifice, His life emanates blessedness and complete harmony. Tuning into His energy by repeating His mantra has a calming and soothing effect on the mind.

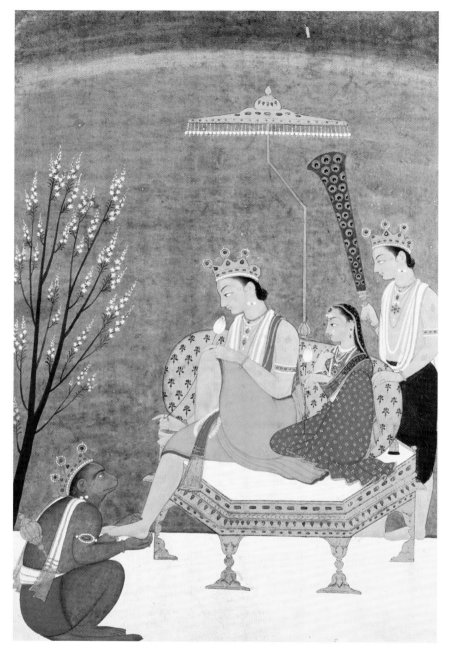

Om Śrī rāmāya namaḥ

ॐ श्री रामाय नमः

OM Sri Durgayai Namah

Prostrations to Mother Durga

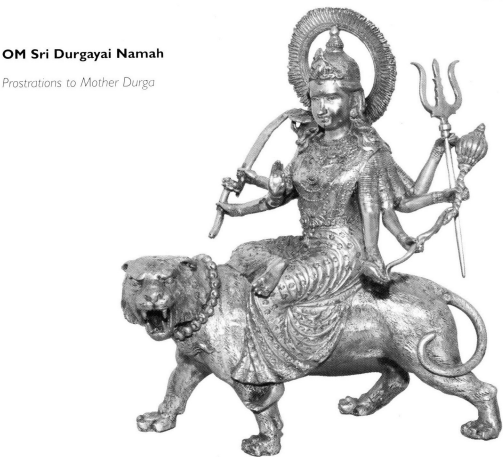

Durga represents the motherhood aspect of the Absolute. She is the force, or *shakti*, through which divinity manifests. Durga is power; She is the protector and benefactor. She is the upholder of *dharma*, righteousness, and is ever ready to fight for the protection of the good. The scriptures say that the consciousness of Brahma, Vishnu, and Siva were united to form the being of Mother Durga. Those who feel reverence for the Mother aspect as divine universal energy feel an affinity with this mantra. She is the perfect teacher, combining in Her personality the firmness and the love necessary to impart knowledge to others successfully.

Om Śrī durgāyai namaḥ

ॐ श्री · दुर्गायै नमः

OM Sri Maha Lakshmyai Namah

Prostrations to the Great Mother Lakshmi

Lakshmi is the ever-bountiful provider. As Vishnu's consort, She aids in the preservation of the universe. She is pictured as a beautiful woman sitting on a lotus blossom with Her arms open in generosity as She confers wealth and prosperity. She bestows both material riches and spiritual abundance. She symbolizes all forms of benevolence, compassion, and goodness. She represents the splendour of the universe, its infinity, and its absolute glory. People with a giving nature who see themselves as channels for all forms of energy, money, knowledge, or love will be attracted to Her.

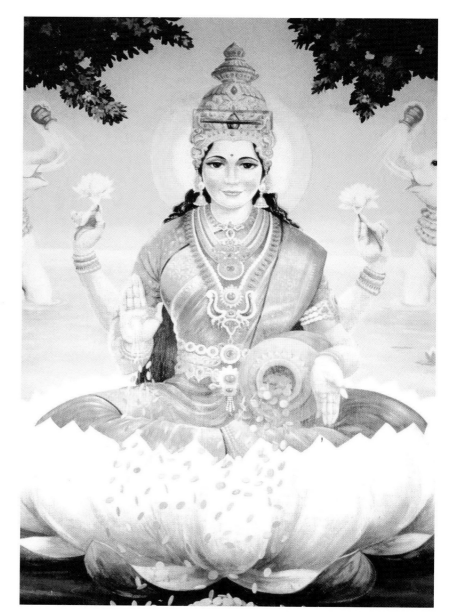

Om Śrī mahālakṣmyai namaḥ

ॐ श्री महालक्ष्म्यै नमः

OM Aim Saraswatyai Namah

Prostrations to Mother Saraswati

Saraswati is the source of all learning and knowledge of the arts and music. Often pictured as a graceful woman dressed in white, She stands for absolute purity. As the consort of Brahma, the creator of the universe, She is also involved with the creation of new things and ideas. Responsible for bestowing wisdom and knowledge, Saraswati is often worshipped by people in the creative field. Repetition of Her mantra bestows intelligence, wisdom, creative achievement, and the power of eloquence.

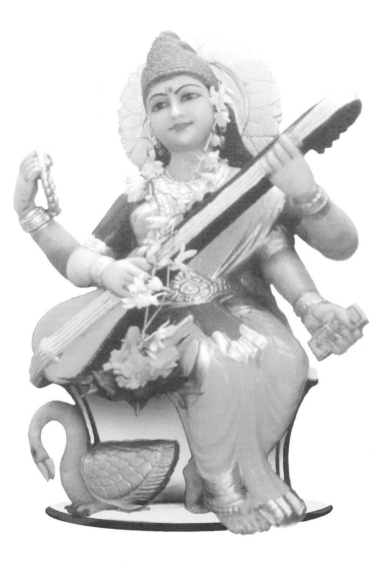

Om aiṃ sarasvatyai namaḥ

ॐ ऐं सरस्वत्यै नमः

OM Sri Hanumate Namah

Prostrations to Blessed Hanuman

Hanuman is the symbol of perfect devotion. He is the greatest and the most selfless devotee of Lord Rama. His total dedication and surrender to Him is the secret behind His extraordinary strength. He presides over *prana*, the vital energy, which bestows on Him great powers. He is also associated with healing. His story is told in the great epic, the *Ramayana*. His mantra has a strong protective energy against any form of negativity or dark influences.

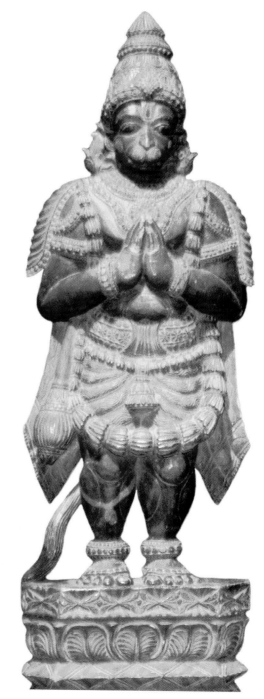

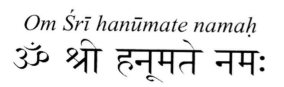

Om Śrī hanūmate namaḥ

ॐ श्री हनूमते नमः

Hare Rama Hare Rama; Rama Rama Hare Hare; Hare Krishna Hare Krishna; Krishna Krishna Hare Hare

My Lord Rama! My Lord Krishna!

Hare rāma hare rāma rāma rāma hare hare
Hare kṛṣṇa hare kṛṣṇa kṛṣṇa kṛṣṇa hare hare

हरे राम हरे राम राम राम हरे हरे
हरे कृष्ण हरे कृष्ण कृष्ण कृष्ण हरे हरे

The repetition of this mantra, called the *maha mantra*, or great mantra, is said to be particularly appropriate to our present age. It invokes the energy of both Rama and Krishna (see pages 88 and 87). Each of these two aspects of the Absolute is a manifestation of the preserving energy of the universe, so together their names give to this mantra a great protective power.

NIRGUNA MANTRAS

Soham

I am That I am

So`haṃ

सोऽहम्

When you repeat this mantra, you focus on your true nature as pure existence itself, without form, without quality, and without past, present, or future. You remember that the body, prana, and mind are your vehicles and do not restrict your consciousness.

OM

OM is the sacred syllable symbolizing absolute consciousness and is the greatest of all mantras. All mantras are contained in OM and all mantras begin with OM. OM is the original vibration; the universe has come from OM, rests in OM, and dissolves in it. AUM, as it is sometimes written, consists of three sounds. "A" is the first sound the vocal apparatus can utter and "M" is the last. In between is the middle range of "U". The three sounds comprising OM therefore encompass all sound. These three sounds signify the three periods of time – past, present, and future – and the three states of consciousness. "A" is the waking state, "U" is the dream state, and "M" is the deep sleep state. All the letters of the Sanskrit alphabet are emanations from OM. All language and thought arise from this word, as do the energy vibrations of the universe itself.

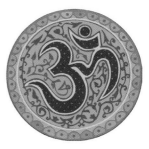

Because of its universal nature, OM can be used as a mantra by those who are unable to find a teacher. However, its very universality and lack of form make it quite difficult for a beginner to grasp. The mind needs to be strong to be able to concentrate on a formless and abstract mantra such as OM.

Japa meditation on OM has a tremendous influence on the mind and body. Vibrations set up by this word are extremely powerful. By holding the hands over the ears and intoning it, you can experience its vibrations on a rudimentary physical level. Correctly pronounced, the sound proceeds from the navel, with a deep and harmonious vibration, and gradually manifests itself at the upper part of the nostrils. As the "U" is pronounced, the sound rolls from the larynx and the root of the tongue right through the palate, the sounding board of the mouth. "M" is the last sound and is produced by closing the lips.

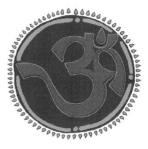

Pronounced merely as spelled, OM has a certain effect upon the nervous system and will benefit the psyche. Pronounced as AUM with concentration and devotion, it arouses and transforms every atom in the physical body, setting up new vibrations and awakening

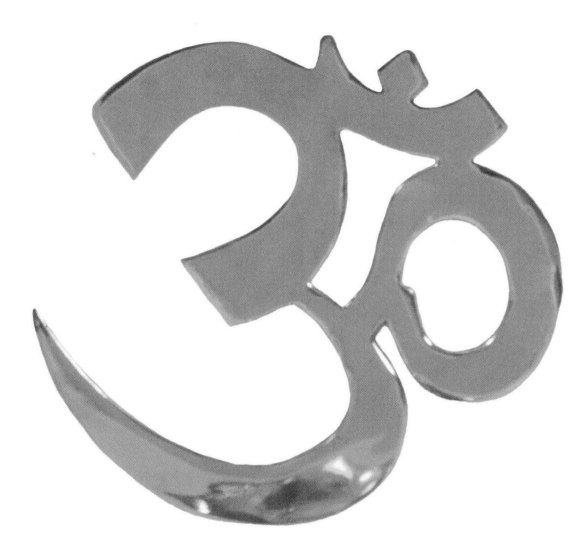

dormant physical and mental powers. It instils vigour and strength in the body. When you feel depressed, chant OM fifty times. You will feel uplifted and joyful. The rhythmic pronunciation of OM makes the mind serene and one-pointed. It brings inspiration and intuition. Swami Sivananda says: "Live in OM. Meditate on OM. Inhale and exhale on OM. Rest peacefully in OM. Take shelter in OM."

CHAPTER SIX

THE TRANSFORMING POWER OF MEDITATION

The gradual progress in physical and mental wellbeing that comes when you meditate is mostly silent and unseen, like the quiet unfolding of a bud into a flower. Try not to set up expectations or goals for change as it may well discourage you if you feel you do not reach them within a certain time. Changes occur at deep and subtle levels, and only gradually will they reveal themselves either to you or to the outside world. There are no objective tests to measure your progress in meditation. However there are universal indicators that all those who meditate on a regular basis will experience sooner or later.

MEDITATION, A GREAT ENERGIZER

Meditation is a vigorous tonic to the physical system. Only recently have scientists become aware of the relationship between the mind and the body cells. Until a few years ago they reacted with total scepticism to yogic demonstrations of mental control over functions such as heartbeat, respiration, and circulation, which are supposedly involuntary. The autonomic nervous system was believed to be independent of any conscious mental process. Now bio-feedback techniques prove that most bodily functions can be controlled by concentration. Modern research substantiates the fact that the mind can control the activity of a single cell, as well as groups of cells.

Each of the body cells is governed by the instinctive, subconscious mind. Each has both individual and collective consciousness. When thoughts and desires pour into the body, the cells are activated, and the body obeys the group demand. During meditation there is generally a tremendous acceleration of prana to the individual cells, rejuvenating them and retarding decay. The powerful soothing waves penetrate the cells and exercise a benign influence on all its organs, setting in motion a process of healing and strengthening that prevents and cures many diseases. It is an established fact that those

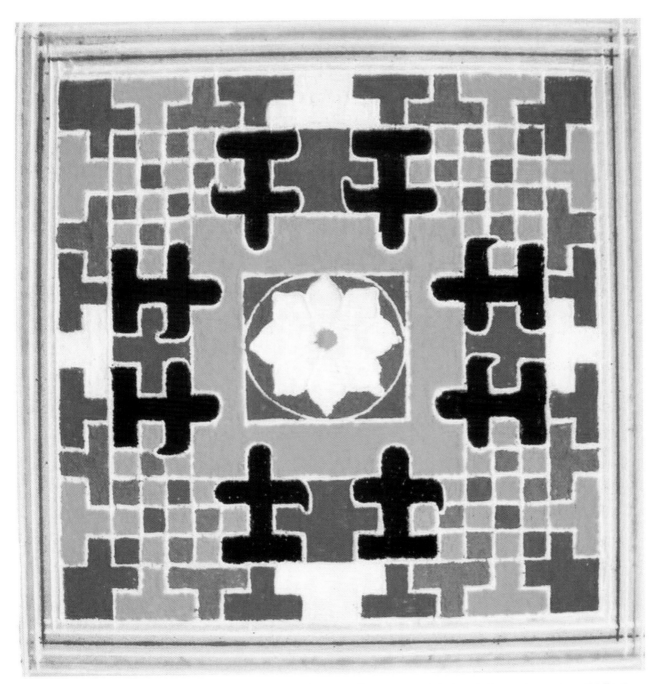

A Siva yantra in coloured sand. A yantra is the deity in the form of a geometrical design and is used as a powerful focal point of concentration and devotion in advanced meditation practice.

who meditate on a regular basis visit the doctor and hospital far less often than those who do not practise.

Meditation helps to prolong the body's anabolic process of cell production, growth, and repair and to reduce the catabolic process of decay. After the age of thirty-five our brain cells die off at a rate of 100,000 a day; meditation reduces this decline, preventing or minimizing senility.

Once you meditate, the time you normally devote to sleep can gradually be reduced; advanced meditators can sleep for as little as three hours a night and still feel more rested and peaceful than before. You will develop a powerful digestive system, with reduced food intake and scanty excretions; you will enjoy a lightness of the body and mind. Your senses will sharpen, resulting in heightened perception and the ability to hear sounds and see objects more clearly and at a more subtle level. Meditation is a great energizer. You will feel newly alive, full of vigour and vitality. Sparkling eyes with a steady gaze, a beautiful complexion, a powerful but sweet voice, and a strong, sweet-smelling and healthy body will tell you that your meditation is proceeding well.

ACHIEVING CALMNESS OF MIND

By decreasing the heart rate and consumption of oxygen, meditation greatly reduces stress levels and acts as a powerful tonic not only to the body but also to the nervous system. Each part of the body, down to the individual cells, is allowed to relax and rejuvenate. Real progress in your practice is accurately measured by the peacefulness, serenity, and calmness that you demonstrate in the waking state. Does your mind seem to be shedding a little of its dullness or heaviness? Do you feel more peaceful, happier with yourself, and less prone to emotional outbursts? Are serenity of mind and a sense of contentment starting to flourish? If the answer to any of these questions is yes, then you will know that you are advancing in your practice.

You will become aware that you identify closely with emotions, thoughts, and actions and you will gradually move away from this, assuming the role of witness, as if you were watching someone else. By observing yourself without judgement or praise, you will lessen the controlling power of your habitual thoughts and emotions. In detaching from the games of the ego, you will learn how to take responsibility for yourself. If you suffer from addictions of any kind, you will find that your cravings for the addictive substance or action will gradually start to fade. Attachments, likes and dislikes, and their accompanying restlessness and agitation of mind will diminish. Negative tendencies will decrease and your mind will become steadier; your face will be calm and serene. Balance and self-composure, harmony, happiness, and satisfaction with life will establish themselves. You will have an unruffled mind. You will be calm, tranquil, and poised.

THE DEVELOPMENT OF INNER CLARITY

Along with mental strength comes a corresponding expansion in the power of your intellect. The practice of concentration increases willpower and memory, resulting in a sharp and bright intellect. Alacrity, acumen, and agility will slowly broaden your capacity to turn out tremendous work. Your ability to clarify ideas and remove doubts will develop and as a consequence you will become skillful in making correct and speedy decisions. What used to take four hours will take only one. What was cloudy and hazy before will become clear and definite; what was difficult before will come more easily; and what was complex, bewildering, and confusing will be grasped effortlessly. You will work with scientific accuracy and great efficiency. You will have a one-pointed, clear, strong, subtle mind, with mental images clear-cut and with thoughts well defined and well grounded. You will discriminate and detach from the trammels of day-to-day living, resulting in less stress and more peace.

THE GRADUAL TRANSFORMATION OF THE PERSONALITY

As a result of this new-found peace, you will experience a changed view of the universe and develop different patterns of behaviour. Lethargy and laziness, pain, and sorrow will decrease and in their place cheerfulness and joy will grow. Because your attention to what you do as you do it will increase, you will find you live more in the present. The time you spend in dreaming of an imaginary future or of an exaggerated past will lessen. You will find that you remove clutter from your life. Within a few weeks of starting to practise, most meditators clear out drawers, cupboards, and files. You will attack – with gusto – jobs and tasks that have been waiting for you for many months. Instead of being piled high, your pending file at work will seldom be full.

As you advance in your practice, you will gradually develop a love for all, even for those who despise you. Your strength of mind will allow you to bear insult and injury and to meet the challenges of everyday life with energy, fortitude, and patience. Situations and people that previously upset you will now no longer do so. The computers will still break down, the traffic will still grind to a halt, the boss will still put you under pressure, but you will find that you are less affected by the turmoil, keeping a cool head and a balanced mind when before you were stressed, angry, and anxious. You will develop a magnetic and dynamic personality. Those who come into contact with you will be influenced by your inspiring and more compassionate behaviour, powerful speech, and spiritual nature. People will draw joy, peace, and strength from you. You will attract people to you and lift their mood and minds.

Of course, these signs of progress will not manifest immediately, and you may require many years of regular practice before you start to reap some of the more profound benefits outlined. Do not grow dejected with the idea that you are not making headway.

Sometimes the progress will be imperceptible. However, even after a month or two you will start to see improvements in your life at all levels. Your friends and family will ask whether you have been on holiday or have taken some cure! When these changes do start to appear, try not to become complacent and curtail your practice. Do not become self-satisfied. This is so important. As we pointed out earlier, the layers of impurities in the mind run deep and it is only when you start to work on them that you realize how many there are. If you conquer one obstacle, another obstacle will be ready to manifest. If you control a craving for taste, you may find another craving develops with doubled force to assail you. If you remove greed, anger may appear more forcefully than before. If you drive egoism out of one door, it enters through another.

Great patience, perseverance, vigilance, and undaunted strength are needed. Be firm, steady, and steadfast. People may mock you. Be silent. People may insult you; be silent. Every temptation that is resisted, every destructive thought that is curbed, every desire that is subdued, every angry word that is withheld, every noble aspiration that is encouraged, every sublime idea that is cultivated adds to the growth of willpower, good character, and inner peace. You will engage in rich and rewarding relationships as you learn to understand yourself and others better; you will experience a full and well-lived life as you take control in ways that previously seemed impossible. Meditation paves the way for perfection; continue your practice and reap the beauty of peace and stillness that will slowly unfold within.

AS YOU ADVANCE

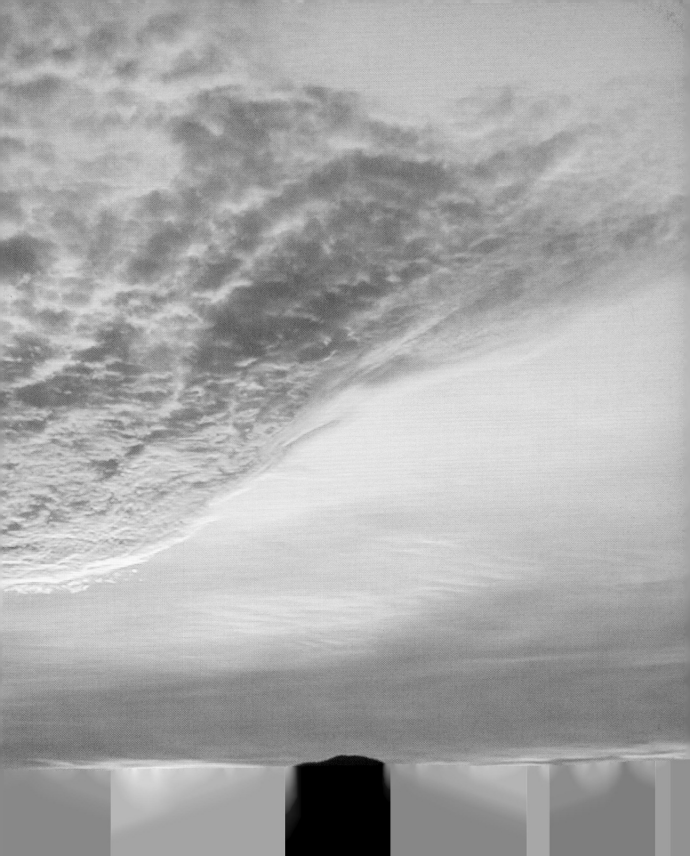

CHAPTER SEVEN

DEVOTIONAL AND VEDANTIC MEDITATION

The essence of meditation is simple: to sustain concentration on a single object. The beginner can focus on any object of an uplifting nature, a sacred sound being one of the easiest ways to gather the ever-wandering rays of the mind. At the outset of our practice, we are unaware of the powers of a mantra, feeling only the relaxing effects produced by its repetition. We do not tend to connect to it with the heart. However, as we deepen the practice, the awareness will gradually dawn that there is more to the mantra. As our minds start to quieten through regular practice and a more balanced and healthy lifestyle, our inner understanding will become more refined. As the mind is freed from negativity, meditation will become more meaningful and rewarding. Progress will manifest as a new sense of connection to the mantra on the heart level and a clearer sense of our true identity.

DEVOTIONAL MEDITATION

Developing devotion through mantra repetition opens the heart and is a key to success in meditation. You must put your heart into your practice, otherwise it will remain superficial and will not bring deep healing to your mind. In the *Yoga Sutras* Patanjali writes that concentration should be practised for a long time, without interruption, and with sincere devotion. Devotional meditation – also called *saguna* meditation – involves visualizing the form of an aspect of the supreme reality and repeating his or her name by means of a devotional or saguna mantra. It is this repetition that will bring you to develop a relationship with God, the Absolute.

The supreme reality is not limited to a specific form, yet He can take all possible forms. When He takes form He becomes personal. When you take a saguna mantra you are associating with *bhakti yoga*, the path of yoga that transforms emotions into universal love. Bhakti yoga centres on a personal form of the supreme essence to give a focus for and to develop our devotion.

ARATI

To purify the energy in your meditation area, you can use a short ritual called *arati* at the end of each meditation session. This is a ceremony in which a flame is offered in your place of meditation while mantras are repeated. If you are travelling and have to meditate in a different place for a period of time, try to perform arati before meditating as it clears the space of any negative energies. As you become familiar with meditation practice and with the energy changes it brings about, you find you want to strengthen this purity within and around you. Arati will help a great deal in this. The text of the arati used at the Sivananda Yoga Centres is on page 159.

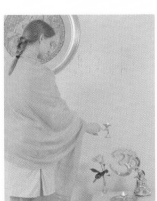

Bhakti yoga teaches us how to develop this personal relationship with the supreme essence. It is the approach to self-realization through pure love, which is poured upon the chosen deity or aspect of God. It gives us complete freedom as to which form we want to relate to and the nature of the relationship itself. God is not only He, the Divine Father, but is also She, the Divine Mother. We can relate to God as a friend, as lord, as a divine child, or as the divine beloved. In the bhakti yogic tradition we see God as the lord of this universe (*ishvara*), in his triple action of creation, preservation, and destruction. The three aspects of God engaged in these three cosmic activities are called Brahma, Vishnu, and Siva. The power of creation is also represented as a feminine form, the Divine Mother, the carrier of life, the caretaker of all beings in the universe. The power of preservation is best represented in an avatar or divine incarnation, in which God manifests in a form on earth to restore righteousness and preserve balance and peace. Krishna, Buddha, and Christ are all regarded as avatars, and Christianity is one example of the bhakti path. The destructive or transformative aspect of God is usually represented by Lord Siva, whose cosmic dance symbolizes the eternal dance of the energy in the universe, energy that continually transforms all manifestations, destroying before it can be recreated.

Besides mantra repetition there are other practices that help to develop devotion: rituals like offerings of flowers or *arati* (see left), or prayers to a chosen aspect of God. With time, the feeling of connection with God will grow stronger. You will become less dependent on your emotional relationship with others for your balance and happiness, since your relationship with God will give you much satisfaction and joy. True devotion will carry you through the emotional ups and downs of life and will be the anchor you can hang on to at times of major challenges. It will also help to steady your mind and develop concentration. The mind follows the heart, so you will find it easy to focus on something for which you have love. Meditating on your *ishta devata* (chosen aspect of God) is the

first step of this devotional approach to union with the supreme essence. Eventually, you realize that this form is none other than your inner Self and will see the Self in all forms. In this sense, the form does not limit your consciousness, but takes you to infinite consciousness. You may wonder why it is then necessary to use a form of God in your meditation practice. The reason is that as long as the heart is not awakened, it is not possible to steady the mind. Developing devotion is not a detour; it is a necessary step in the meditation process.

Bija mantras

Some saguna mantras do not focus on a personal form of the Divine, but connect you to the supreme reality through the pure mystical power of sound. They are called *bija*, or seed, mantras. They have no intellectual meaning. They work by acting directly on the *nadis*, the nerve tubes of the astral body. Vibrating in the chakras along the spine, acting as a subtle massage, they release blockages and allow the *kundalini energy* (spiritual power) to flow more freely. Just as the various deities are aspects of the one supreme, so the various bija mantras are aspects of the supreme mantra, OM. Bija mantras are seed letters directly derived from the fifty primeval sounds. They generally consist of a single letter, although some are compounded. Every deity has its own seed syllable. Because of their tremendous power, bija mantras are not generally given for initiation. Japa on them may be practised only by those who are in a pure state and their use is preceded by intricate rituals. When improperly repeated, they can actually bring harm to the psychic system. Advanced meditation such as this should be attempted only under the guidance of a teacher.

VEDANTIC MEDITATION

In the practice of vedantic meditation one does not only sit for meditation at a specific time, but applies the meditative process throughout the day. The philisophy of vedanta is based on the teachings of the Upanishads, which form the concluding section of

THE UPANISHADS

The *Upanishads* are the concluding portions of the *Vedas*, and form the foundation on which vedantic philosophy is based. They are considered to be the mystic experiences of the great sages. The word *Upanishad* means "to sit down close to" (one's teacher or guru), referring to the method of transmitting spiritual knowledge orally from guru to disciple. Traditionally 108 *Upanishads* are referred to. Swami Sivananda says of them: "There is no work in the whole world that is so thrilling, soul-stirring, and inspiring as the *Upanishads*. The *Upanishads* teach the philosophy of absolute unity and contain the sublime truths of vedanta. The breadth of vision, the profundity of insight, and the marvellous gamut of inclusiveness revealed in these holy writings are remarkable and breathtaking."

VEDANTA

Vedanta is one of the six classical philosophies of India. Swami Sivananda declared it the ideal to be embodied in life, and yoga the practical means to achieve this goal. Vedanta proclaims that each individual person, in his or her very essence, is identical with the Supreme Being. It reminds each one of us of our true nature. Vedanta states that there is a common Self or common consciousness in all, urging us to forego the sense of individuality or possession, "I-ness", or "my-ness" and identify ourselves with a self-existent, self-luminous Essence, seeing the Self in ourselves and in all beings. Vedanta teaches the unity of life and the oneness of consciousness. It is found in the teachings of the Vedas, the sacred writings of the great sages of India, to whom it was revealed while they were in deep meditation.

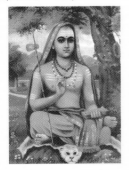

Sri Sankaracharya, who lived around 1,200 years ago, is the main exponent of the philosophy of vedanta.

the *Vedas*, the most ancient scriptural texts of India. (*Vedanta* means literally "the end of the *Vedas*".) The origin of the *Vedas* is unknown, but it is said that they were given through inspiration to the holy men who sat meditating upon God. The philosophy of vedanta states that our true nature is infinite consciousness, the cosmic Self, which is one and the same in all beings. Vedantic meditation is associated with the path of *jnana yoga*, the path of knowledge. It aims at reaching Self-knowledge without the help of a form, but rather through focusing directly on pure consciousness.

The meditative process in the path of jnana yoga aims at realizing this truth first intellectually, then through direct experience. It is based on observation, discrimination, and detachment. It requires spiritual maturity, a balanced personality, and an already calm and strong mind.

There are various vedantic meditation methods for realizing our true identity. All are based on overcoming the identification with our body and mind in order to realize the full extent of our being. Just as a container creates the illusion that the space inside is separate from and smaller than the space outside, so the mind creates its own walls, and the illusion of separation from the Self. Removal of this identification with the form is the very core of vedantic meditation regardless of the method used.

The practice of negation

Neti-neti, meaning "not this, not this," is the method of vedantic analysis by negation. It is the keynote of vedantic inquiry. By finding out what you are not, you move towards an understanding of who or what you are. Through negation of everything that is limited, you exhaust the mental modifications and find the answer to the question *Who am I?* In this type of meditation, you ask yourself the questions: *Am I the body? Am I the prana? Am I the senses? Am I the emotions? Am I the mind?* Each time, you conclude that you are more than this. You are not this limited sense of self; you are not your name, your job, your nationality, or your religion. Finally, worldly

experiences are transcended, for all has been negated and nothing remains but the Self. It is initially the intellect that comes to this conclusion. However, direct experience is necessary, as it is ultimately not a matter of intellectual understanding. When all intellectual possibilities have been negated, you have achieved ninety-nine per cent of your goal. The one hundred per cent mark is when you receive direct intuitive realization.

The practice of observation of the mind

Sakshi bhav consists in adopting the attitude of a witness. You observe the mind as though you are watching a film, but you do not identify with it. Whatever situation you experience throughout the day, your reaction is the same: *I am not involved in this; I am only watching it happen*. It entails introspection and close awareness of all thoughts. The mind does not want to be watched and will slow down, but it does not give up without a struggle. It will try many ways to deceive you, to persuade you to stop watching. Unless you are extremely vigilant, it will constantly divert attention away from itself. You must observe this with patience, then firmly return to the witness state. Gently guide the mind, without fighting it. With the repetition of *OM sakshi aham (I am witness of all my actions)*, and continual disassociation from those actions, the individual ego eventually vanishes.

The practice of absorption

Laya chintana, the practice of absorption, is an advanced method that aims at absorbing the mind back into its very source, pure consciousness. The philosophical basis of this practice is the common identity between the macrocosm and the microcosm. By observing the process of the creation of the universe, you develop an intuitive understanding of how your own mind functions and how to bring it back to its source. In this meditation, the effect is absorbed into its cause. Vedanta states that the whole universe is but a combination of five elements: earth, water, fire, air, and ether. These are found in both the macrocosm and the microcosm that is

the human body. In the process of universal evolution, the five elements manifest from the cosmic source in the following order: ether, air, fire, water, and earth. Laya chintana meditation consists in reversing the process of evolution, or enacting in your consciousness the process of involution: starting with the least subtle element, you move back to the most subtle, merging each into the next.

You first meditate on the earth element and visualize that all solid matter originates in a liquid form (the water element). That liquid state of energy originates in fire. Fire finds its origin in the explosion of gas. Gas or the air element manifests from ether or pure space. Space itself exists only within pure consciousness. This creative visualization process, in which each element is brought back into its cause, finally brings you to the realization of the true nature of your body-mind vehicle. It looks solid, but is made mainly of liquid, behind which is the fire of the metabolic process; further beyond that is the movement of prana, and further still is empty space. Finally you realize that that which contains space is consciousness.

The abstract path

Needless to say the techniques of vedantic meditation are highly advanced and require a thorough preparation of the mind, made pure, selfless, and focused through the practice of selfless service, asanas and pranayama, and the devotional method of meditation. The teachings tell us that before even approaching the jnana yoga path the practice of both raja and bhakti yoga must be well developed. Success in vedantic meditation requires the help of a highly evolved teacher who will guide you away from the tendency to intellectual pride or a feeling of dryness and sterility if the practice is carried out incorrectly. Start by practising saguna meditation to master the emotions, the senses, and the mind, and most importantly to develop humility, before you venture forward on to this abstract path of meditation.

CHAPTER EIGHT

THE ART OF RIGHT LIVING

According to yoga philosophy the universe is governed by a law of cosmic harmony called the *law of dharma*. On an individual level, following your own *dharma* means acting responsibly and behaving in a manner appropriate to your age, your role in society, and your level of spiritual awareness. For success in meditation, this sense of social responsibility and right living must be highly developed. Otherwise, the basic traits of your personality will stay unchanged: the same jealousy, pride, anger, and egoism will continue to dominate your behaviour.

People who have meditated for many years with little progress may complain about the lack of efficacy of meditation. In these cases we frequently find the practice of right living has been neglected. Swami Sivananda says: "He who meditates without ethical perfection cannot get the fruits of meditation."

Many people express surprise at this, especially as it is unpopular nowadays to talk of ethical standards. Why is it necessary to develop a code of ethical conduct along with the practice of meditation? Why should we base our behaviour on principles of right living at all? The answer is because we would not become truly human if we did not do so. Irresponsible and thoughtless action gives rise to unhappiness and sorrow. Right living allows us to rise above the limitations of instinctive life.

However, in the yogic tradition, right living is not the final goal. Its aim is to purify the mind so that we will be fit to receive the knowledge of the soul; so we can spiritualize ourselves gradually by permanently transforming our negativities. Yoga propounds that all existence is in a perpetual state of evolution, in a constant state of development towards a fuller manifestation of the inherent divinity of this existence. The core and purpose of all right living is to lead the way to this achievement via a process of mental purification. This can be reached only by refraining from negative thoughts and

actions, and by simultaneously practising good thoughts and actions. The aim of right living is the elevation of actions, emotions, and aspirations, bringing purity and calmness to the mind. A pure mind becomes one-pointed and moves naturally inwards. The state of meditation will come naturally once the mind is purified.

The philosophical basis of the practice of dharma is that there is only one Self expressing itself in an infinite number of beings. Beyond the diversity of bodies and personalities lies the same consciousness. Existence is common; one life vibrates in all beings. We live truly ethically when we live in the awareness of this oneness with everything. This awareness expands with practice. Ultimately our relationship with people and the environment around us reflects our relationship to ourselves. If we hurt another creature, we hurt ourselves. If we help another person, we help ourselves. The less we are attuned to our body, feelings, and thoughts, the unhappier and more isolated we feel. We feel that we have a separate existence from others and as a result find it difficult to connect with people. To be established in the art of right living is to feel a connectedness with everything on all levels of existence. At one end of the spectrum we perceive diversity, which is to be respected and cherished, and at the other end lies the intuitive realization of the oneness of all things. Right living is the path that leads from diversity to unity.

True morality lies neither in self-assertion, nor in individual efforts for one's own good, but in offering oneself as a contribution to the wellbeing of the whole world. In the yogic tradition this offering is seen as the duty of each and every person. The ideals of duty come before personal rights in a spirit of sacrifice and surrender. This concept of duty to existence in its entirety may seem remote to many of us in the West who are under siege from consumerism to spend much of our lives in the pursuit of pleasure and individual privilege. However, if we diligently take care of what we recognize as our duties, our heart and mind will expand, our comfort and prosperity increase. Our pleasures become more refined; our

happiness, our enjoyments, and recreations become more dignified. Happiness is like a shadow; if pursued it moves away; but if we let it alone and focus with love on our duties, a new sense of inner contentment and harmony will be ours.

The practice of right living broadens the heart and reduces selfishness. However, our behaviour only undergoes a lasting transformation if we work on it constantly and systematically. If we look at our mind as a garden and the impurities as weeds, daily clearing is needed to keep the garden in bloom. We create impressions in the mind by each action we perform. Repeated actions develop into a tendency, the tendency into habit, the habit into character, and the character into destiny. We need to take conscious responsibility for our actions and to develop a keen awareness of their consequences.

The basic practice of right living is to train the mind to give. As Swami Sivananda says: "Giving is the law of life." This attitude can be developed in daily life: giving our time and our energy, sharing food, giving encouragement. Give part of your income to charity. Share your happiness and positivity with others. Keep in front of you Swami Sivananda's injunction: "Do good and be good." The goal of your life is to express your full potential and your true identity. To achieve this goal, instincts need to be sublimated and the higher aspect of your personality needs to be trained to assert itself. This higher part of the mind is strengthened by the performance of selfless actions. Act selflessly with a happy and light frame of mind: a sense of freedom and joy comes with a sincere disregard of personal reward.

Refrain from performing actions that you would not like other people to know about. You will become secretive and unable to relax for fear that you will be discovered. Be aware of the true motive behind each of your actions. The motive is more important than the action itself. Most actions have at their root a subconscious habit, based on the desire for pleasure, security, power, and

recognition. At night, after the day is done, sit down, close your eyes and go back over the day's events. Think what you left undone and what mistakes you made, and with no sense of recrimination or shame, ask yourself what you should have done instead. Use your spiritual diary (see Chapter Nine) to guide you. The practice of regular introspection will help you overcome not only the waves of negative thoughts that can sometimes overwhelm you but also the deeper negative thought patterns in the subconscious mind. As you continue the practice, you will notice that your motives will become selfless and compassionate.

THE RULES OF RIGHT LIVING

The yogic rules of social and personal conduct are called *yamas* and *niyamas*; they are the first two steps of the raja yoga system and the foundation of spiritual life on which the superstructure of meditation is built. Yamas and niyamas annihilate desires, cravings, and negative qualities, removing harshness, violence, and cruelty from the personality. Their practice will gradually melt the heart and fill it with love, kindness, and goodness.

Yamas

The yamas are five practices that allow us to relate to the outside world in the right way. They are rules of social conduct akin to the Ten Commandments of Christianity or the Eight-Fold Path of Buddhism. They are *ahimsa* (non-violence); *satya* (truthfulness); *brahmacharya* (control of the senses); *asteya* (non-stealing), and *aparigraha* (non-possessiveness).

Ahimsa (non-violence) Ahimsa is to abstain from harm to any living creature, in thought, word, and deed. It does not mean merely non-injury or non-violence but also perfect harmlessness and an active practice of love. Ahimsa includes forgiveness, mercy, and protection of other beings, especially those who are weaker. It embraces compassion, charitable acts, and kindness, purifying and softening the heart.

You break the practice of ahimsa by showing contempt, by entertaining prejudice against someone, by gossiping, by harbouring thoughts of hatred and anger, by lying, by failing to relieve pain or trouble, or by approving of another's harsh action. In all its forms, violence is an enemy of wisdom. It results only in pain and sorrow. It separates and divides. One harsh word can destroy the relationship of people who have been united in love for many years. Violence against another is the main cause of mental restlessness. If the thought of violence vibrates in your mind, it brings distortion and prompts you to do more harm. Try to safeguard every living being as best you can; feel compassion when you see someone in pain, relieve suffering if you can. Stoically bear insult, criticism, and rebuke. Do not retaliate. Hold anger against no one. Forgive all.

Satya (truthfulness) The practice of truthfulness will make the mind peaceful, clear, and able to see the truth, which is the essence of being. It includes self-restraint, absence of jealousy, forgiveness, courage, patience, endurance, kindness, and love. It will free you from the habit of worrying. Your thoughts should agree with your words and your words with your actions. Many people think one thing, say another, and do yet another, leading to distrust and animosity. Be gentle with the truth. If speaking the truth causes injury or pain, it is no longer a virtue; brutal honesty is not truthfulness. Untruth includes exaggeration, lying, vanity, conceit, pretension, and breaking promises. It brings tension, worry, and apprehension — the deep-seated fear that dishonesty will be discovered. Remember that you seldom lie just once. One lie often leads to another in an endless succession of deceit, dulling your conscience and poisoning your subconscious mind. You soon become overwhelmed with restless thoughts making meditation impossible. A person who is truthful is very powerful. Swami Sivananda says: "Have ceaseless devotion to truth. Be ready to sacrifice your all for it. You will soon become a great soul."

OJAS

Ojas is the subtle essence that produces our vitality. It is present in every cell of the body and is the foundation of physical immunity, maintaining the natural resistance of all bodily tissue. It sustains the lifespan of each cell and fights against aging, decay, and disease. A person with strong ojas is rarely ill, and is compassionate, creative, loving, and peaceful.

To increase ojas soak ten almonds overnight in water. In the morning peel the almonds and place them in a blender with a cup of warm milk. Add a pinch of cardamom powder and freshly ground black pepper and one teaspoonful of honey. Blend for a couple of minutes. Drink immediately.

Brahmacharya (control of the senses) Often equated with celibacy, in reality brahmacharya refers to the control of all the senses. However, it is not sensual suppression, but the channelling of energy for the purposes of deep meditation.

The most powerful impulse in nature, after breathing, is procreation. The pull to sexual union is so strong that it often overpowers all wisdom and reason. Cosmic energy, which forms and perpetuates the galaxies and the world, is the same energy that is continuously vibrating in the body and mind. This life energy, or universal prana, manifests on the gross physical level as sexual energy. Sexual and sensual energy, when properly channelled, transform into *ojas*, a subtle and spiritual energy that is stored in the body, and in particular in the brain.

Ojas is the creative power, the vital energy, and the vigour in a person who has converted sensuality into spirituality. In the sexual experience, this energy is dissipated and lost. But through the practice of brahmacharaya, this same energy is preserved. A person who has an abundance of ojas has a magnetic personality, lustrous face, strong voice, high level of vitality and health, and a powerful ability to concentrate. When this energy is out of balance, you will find greed, passion, too much talking, too much sleep, tiredness, irritability, and an inability to focus.

Celibacy is a difficult concept fully to understand, and one that is quite foreign to the Western mind, but it is an ancient and timeless practice of all spiritual traditions of the world. Each tradition has its group of aspirants who have renounced worldly desires and sensual pleasures. In the yogic tradition monks and nuns are known as *swamis* or *sannyasins*.

But celibacy is not recommended for all as the sexual instinct is so powerful, and common sense needs to be applied, taking into account your age, condition, and depth of commitment to a spiritual life. Brahmacharya does not necessarily mean full celibacy, but an understanding of the purpose of channelling sensual energy to

develop mental power. It can be practised by having a more regulated sex life, avoiding excess, and turning the mind to find joy through other avenues, particularly through spiritual practices such as selfless service, spiritual chanting, prayer, and meditation.

Asteya (non-stealing) Stealing means taking what does not belong to you, and includes taking credit for others' actions. The desire for other people's possessions will rob you of your peace of mind. Asteya includes overcoming greed and the tendency to waste. Stealing in any form is a result of greed. Hoarding money, eating too much, wasting resources, or even somebody's time, keeping or taking more than is needed are all forms of stealing. Anything done with a view to concealing it from others is considered to be theft, as is not sharing what we have. Stealing dulls the conscience, and brings guilt, dishonour, and an increase in desires. Be honest in all dealings and earn only by your own effort.

Aparigraha (non-possessiveness) Aparigraha means overcoming the greed for possessing objects. It is similar to asteya, though there is a subtle difference between the two. *Steya* (stealing) is the effect of a wrong understanding of life, expressed in wrong action. *Parigraha* (possessiveness) is the real cause of greed. It is a thirsting for attention and recognition, for other people's property, and for reward. It is based on ignorance of the laws of life, which teach us that we are all part of one existence and that as a consequence we need to give. It does not mean giving away all our possessions. However, we should not accumulate things unnecessarily. Having too many possessions creates attachment, which in turn creates fear of loss, anger, and jealousy. Aparigraha also means not accepting gifts if they lead to luxury, bribery, or manipulation. Its practice is an aid to non-violence, truthfulness and non-stealing. It removes fear and attachment, brings contentment, and gives clarity to the mind and a purpose to life. Practice generosity, give abundantly, and live selflessly.

SATSANG

Satsang, literally translated as "association with the wise" is considered to be one of the most powerful ways of imbibing and absorbing spiritual knowledge. Satsang can be a gathering in a church, synagogue, temple, meeting house, or in someone's home – anywhere where prayer and meditation are practised and where the words or presence of saints and sages prevail. When people gather together to listen to spiritual discourse or writings, to pray, or to meditate, a potent vibration is set up, highly beneficial to all present. The process brings peace and contentment, expanding the heart and opening the mind. In the East people are advised to seek the company of holy men and women and listen to their conversation and advice. The strength and energy that is transmitted when listening to or being in the presence of such people, or reading spiritual writings, is immeasurable.

Niyamas

The practice of yamas purifies the mind and establishes right relationship with the outside world; niyamas are rules of individual behaviour. Niyamas weed out negativity and implant virtues, freeing the mind from the influence of anger, pride, passion, jealousy, greed, and delusion. Niyamas regulate habits and strengthen willpower, preparing the mind for meditation. The niyamas are *saucha* (purity of body and environment), *santosha* (contentment), *tapas* (austerity), *svadhyaya* (the study of spiritual writings), and *ishvara pranidhana* (surrender to the Divine will).

Saucha (purity) Saucha starts with physical purity such as keeping your surroundings clean, bathing regularly, and taking care of the body by exercising, eating pure food, and wearing clean clothes. Mental purity is practised through selfless service, releasing negative emotions and thoughts, developing good qualities, *japa* (repetition of mantras), and *satsang* (the company of spiritually-minded people, see left). The practice of saucha helps to remove jealousy, worry, the habit of gossiping, and anger. Joyfulness, contentment, serenity and harmony, kindness, and patience are all manifestations of purity.

Santosha (contentment) Contentment and real happiness are not found in outer objects but within. Contentment brings peace and fullness of life. It means accepting life as it comes, and being happy with whatever conditions arise. Only when your mind is freed from the pressures of desire and frustration can it be integrated and purified. With this purity comes cheerfulness. When you are content you neither complain, nor crave what you don't have, and you are free from what other people think or say about you. All sense of comparison, rivalry, and jealousy arises from a feeling of discontent. Discontent poisons your life. A distracted mind is always discontented, and will constantly seek entertainment in outer objects. It will be prey to jealousy, gossip, and back-biting. Judge your success in life not on the basis of what you possess, your position, or your intelligence, but rather on the freedom you have from desires and cravings.

Tapas (austerity) Tapas is doing those things which are difficult and avoiding doing those things which are easy, in order to strengthen the mind. The mind is like a muscle. A muscle only strengthens when it works against itself. Similarly the mind must be made to work to develop strength. There are three forms of tapas: physical, verbal, and mental. Fasting, withstanding physical difficulties, and bearing discomfort are austerities of the body. The practice of silence (*mouna*) and speaking only constructive and truthful words constitute verbal tapas. Changing negative thoughts to positive, conquering anger and hatred, not complaining, bearing insult and injury, and the practice of serenity are all forms of mental tapas. Facing life with all its imperfections, limitations, and shortcomings with understanding and faith is great tapas. Meditation is the highest form of tapas. The benefits are immeasurable and include good health, concentration, endurance, and strong willpower.

Svadhyaya (the study of spiritual writings) When you read spiritual writings, you tune into the author's own knowledge and wisdom. The words can act as close companions and are ideal teachers in difficult times. Read spiritual works written by saints or holy men and women to help you keep your spiritual interest alive and feed your mind with positive ideas. Choose an uplifting work and try to understand fully what you have read and put it into daily practice. Svadhyaya also includes repeating mantras. This practice elevates the mind, clears doubts, and weeds out negative thoughts. It creates new, spiritual impressions, and helps concentration, encouraging and strengthening your faith and filling the mind with purity.

Ishwara pranidhana (self-surrender) The literal meaning of ishwara pranidhana is "placing oneself in God". It is the practice of devotion. The repetition of mantras, prayer, and the study of devotional books constitute ishwara pranidhana. Honouring God, talking about Him, living for Him, and offering the effects of all actions to Him are all practices in surrender. Surrender draws grace through which intuition develops. The greater the surrender, the greater the ability to perform spiritual practice. When you dedicate all actions to this

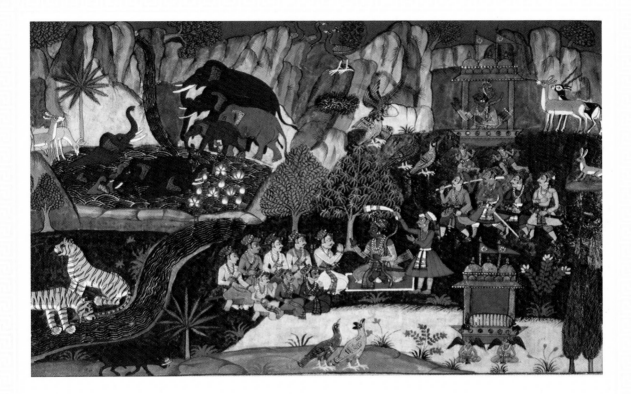

YOGA WRITINGS

The knowledge on which yoga is based has its origins in the great Sanskrit scriptures known as the *Vedas*, works that are considered to have been revealed to the great sages of thousands of years ago. They consequently have no authorship ascribed to them. The four *Vedas* are the *Rig Veda*, the *Atharva Veda*, the *Yajur Veda*, and the *Sama Veda*. They represent the spiritual experiences and knowledge imparted to the rishis (seers) in deep meditation.

One section of the *Vedas* is known as the *Upanishads* (see page 106). Next in importance to the *Vedas* come four works known collectively as the *Itihasas*. These are the *Ramayana*, the *Mahabharata*, the *Yogavasishta,* and the *Harivamsa*. These four works embody all the knowledge contained in the *Vedas* but in a more accessible form. Here are historical narratives, stories and dialogues, analogies, and parables relaying in an easily absorbed manner the foundations of the philosophy, religion, law, duty, morality, and polity

of the yogic tradition. The miniature above shows a scene from the *Ramayana*. The *Bhagavad Gita* (see page 32) is contained within the *Mahabharata*. Other great yogic writings include the *Brahma Sutras*, the *Srimad Bhagavatam*, Sankaracharya's *Viveka Chudamani,* and Patanjali's *Yoga Sutras* (see page 26). Reading these classic works uplifts the mind and is considered to be "indirect satsang" in which the reader can commune with the mind of the author, receiving inspiration and guidance.

inner essence, you will feel protected and guided in life. With practice, surrender becomes unconditional and you will experience profound peace and freedom.

DETACHMENT

Free from attachment, not egotistical,
endowed with firmness and enthusiasm,
unaffected in success and failure,
that person is called pure.

BHAGAVAD GITA XVIII-26

Action performed as duty,
without attachment, without love or hate,
without desire for fruit, is called pure.

BHAGAVAD GITA XVIII-23

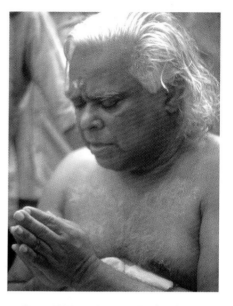

Swami Vishnu-devananda deeply devotional in prayer during satsang

In order to meditate successfully, we need to free our mind from attachment to day-to-day actions and concerns and from their effects, whether good or bad. This is the practice of detachment or non-attachment, and a state of dispassion towards what we do and what we own. It is a mental state that can be developed through the awareness that possession brings with it the fear of loss; and that possession carries within itself pain and selfishness. Actions and possessions in themselves do not bring unhappiness, but our attachment to them and identification with them bring worry and anxiety. Detachment does not mean a shirking of duties, of responsibilities, or of work, nor does it mean owning nothing. It implies the freedom of allowing actions and possessions to be as they are without ownership or "doership" attaching to them. Just as water remains unaffected on a lotus leaf or oil floats on water without being affected in any way, so also should we be in the

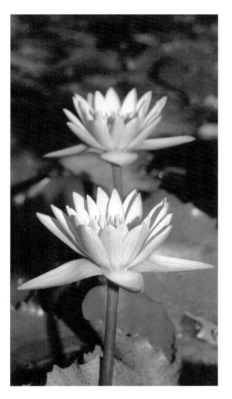

Approach work the way water rolls off the leaf of the lotus, unattached and unaffected.

world unaffected by troubles and difficulties as well as pleasures. If we identify with our actions in our daily life, then these same activities will continue even when we sit still for meditation. Our eyes may be closed, but our minds will be restless. We will find ourselves entangled with thoughts of the office, home, friends, and family. As detachment increases, it is easier to disassociate from our activities when we meditate, and the mind remains unperturbed; it will have been trained to focus inwardly at all times.

One of the most powerful ways to learn detachment is through the practice of *karma yoga*, or selfless service; detachment is learned fully only when we have learned to serve. A karma yogi knows the secret of work: to perform work for work's sake without any motive, and for the sake of the common good in a spirit of sacrifice, with neither attachment nor egoism. The success the karma yogi expects from work is the work itself. Work becomes worship; work becomes meditation.

Karma yoga has several approaches to work that incorporate the spirit of selfless service, each requiring an attitude that initially may be hard to grasp, but with practice becomes rewarding and joyful. The first way is that of equanimity, characterized by tolerance and patience, by an absence of any feeling of grudge, remorse, or resentment. It is working without thinking that the work that we may be doing is beneath us. On the other hand, we should not expand with pride because of the type of work we are doing. Try not to say to yourself: *I have helped this person.* Feel instead: *This person has given me the opportunity to serve. I am thankful.*

Equanimity is having the ability to leave a task without regret and without the feeling of ownership. It is a refusal to accommodate the feeling *I will do this, I won't do that.* It is being able to move from one task to another without grumbling or feeling hard done-by. The great Mahatma Gandhi never differentiated between menial service and "dignified" work. The cleaning of latrines was for him the highest work. Many highly educated persons joined his ashram

to learn yoga thinking he would teach them privately and were severely disappointed when they were asked to clean the latrines first. They immediately left the ashram! Gandhi repaired his own shoes, ground his own flour, spun his own cloth, and did the work of others when they were unable to do their allotted share.

The second way to learn detachment is to look upon yourself as merely an instrument of a higher power; to consider that you are only an agent in whatever you do. This path is characterized by the surrender of the will, and the dedication of all actions to this higher power. Be aware that a higher power is in the heart of every one of us, and when you serve others you are in fact serving this higher power directly. In this light, all actions become sacred.

The third route to detachment is to work without expectation of reward, without expectation of thanks, without motive. Most people work for money, for fame, for position, or for power. Do you expect anything from a baby if you do something for it? Try to work for others without thought of personal gain. Work unselfishly and with disinterest, taking delight in serving others whether they are your employer, your family, or your friends. Try not to expect even the return of love, appreciation, gratitude, or admiration from the people whom you serve or for whom you work.

To work in this way without attachment is without doubt a difficult practice. But the rewards are immense. By working selflessly you purify and expand the heart; you develop inner strength; your spirit of self-sacrifice grows, and there is a corresponding eradication of selfishness; you develop humility; conceit and pride diminish. Pure love, sympathy, tolerance, and mercy grow, along with an expansion and broadening of your outlook on life.

Try to develop enthusiasm for selfless service. Karma yoga requires a willing heart to serve humanity. Be kind to all. Love all. Serve all. Be tolerant and generous towards all. Always scrutinize your motives when you work to check they are pure. Try not to work in a careless, half-hearted manner, hastily and with no interest in what

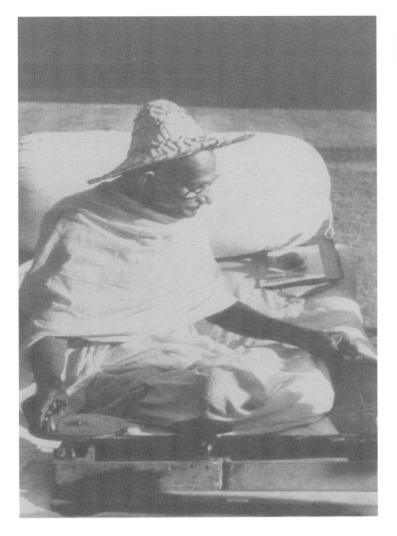

Gandhi weaving, a study of humility and reverence

you do. Take responsibility for all your actions, focusing steadily on the work until completed. The whole heart, mind, and intellect should be in the work; only then can you call it selfless. Create opportunities to serve. Cheer up someone in distress, encourage someone who is depressed, wipe the tears of those in pain, remove sorrow by loving words, make someone smile when there is despair. Karma yoga is the foundation on which meditation is built; no meditation is possible without it.

CHAPTER NINE

SPIRITUAL GUIDANCE

When we start to practise meditation, we are often unaware of the nature of the work we are embarking on. It is only when clarity of mind begins to develop and our consciousness has expanded a little that we realize the need for direction, advice, instruction, and training. Keeping a spiritual diary charts our personal development, acting as both touchstone and encouragement. Finding a spiritual teacher who will support our endeavours and clarify the way ahead enables us to progress with greater confidence towards our goal.

KEEPING A SPIRITUAL DIARY

As meditation practice progresses, you will find that awareness of your moods, emotions, thoughts, and actions increases appreciably. You begin to realize that the knowledge you previously had of your character and personality was considerably distorted by your own clouded perceptions. Most of us are masters at analysing, judging, and criticizing other people's behaviour and character. We see very clearly their failings and shortcomings and — when we are feeling generous — their abilities and gifts, but when we scrutinize our own minds, a veil of ignorance and denial seems to descend.

Even after a short time of regular practice, meditation brings an ability to witness our own behaviour (and along with it, a desire to change). In the beginning this can be quite overwhelming. We start to realize how angry we are, how much time we spend worrying, how tense we feel, how jealous, how greedy... the revelations can be both bewildering and confusing. It is quite common for people to report that they feel less easy after a few months of meditation than they did before they began the practice. Invariably we are not happy with much of what confronts us. There is no need to worry. This is a sign of progress. All great spiritual traditions recognize this stage and offer a means of working with and through the revelations so that they do not overwhelm us, throwing us into depression and despair.

This means is achieved through a spiritual diary, a daily record of our own behavioural patterns, our character traits, and our idiosyncrasies. Keeping a spiritual diary heightens our awareness a hundredfold, allowing us to deal with problems, character defects, and bad habits in a systematic and highly efficient, but nevertheless compassionate manner. A spiritual diary, kept only for yourself or for your spiritual teacher if you have one, acts as a formidable teacher in itself. We start to recognize patterns in our behaviour that we did not know existed. We realize that things we thought we did, we don't do, and things we thought we didn't do, we do. So many of us have been surprised at how irregular our patterns of living are. On a fundamental level we can discover how erratic and detrimental our eating and sleeping habits are to our wellbeing. More surprising still are the subtle and hidden behavioural habits that we start to notice after even just a few months of keeping the diary.

The spiritual diary helps develop the practice of truthfulness, as we slowly learn to monitor in detail and with all honesty the mistakes we make in the course of each day. We expend much energy in concealing our defects, and the diary allows us to confront them in security and privacy. This first step of "confrontation" or discovery is essential in becoming more compassionate and forgiving towards ourselves and, as a natural extension of this, towards other people.

The diary acts as a deterrent to negative actions or thoughts and a reminder to keep on the right path. If you know you will have to record it in your diary later, you may not take that extra piece of chocolate, that drink, that cigarette, or you may resist being irritated by a situation or jealous of someone.

The diary encourages us to keep our practice steady. It reminds us that time is passing and that each day is the day to start life anew. It reminds to bring a rhythm and regularity into our daily routine and to our spiritual practice.

To start your own diary, we suggest that you work on issues you feel you can tackle with relative ease. Swami Sivananda stresses the

importance of being detailed in our analysis and working only on those details. If we look after the smaller points, the strength will develop to tackle bigger problems that may present themselves in the future. Avoid setting yourself visionary goals that are virtually unattainable; it is much better to establish small objectives and work with determination towards them. In this way, you minimize the possibility of abandoning them altogether. Not only that, you will find your willpower and inner strength will markedly improve. You can expand the scope of your diary as you progress.

Progress

Along with the removal of shortcomings, start to monitor how you develop good character. Practise courage, honesty, contentment, joy, or laughter on a daily basis. Swami Sivananda recommends taking one positive quality a month and working to increase it gradually. For example, documenting them each night in your diary, try doing three acts of kindness a day for a month, or feeling grateful five times a day for a month, or being cheerful four times a day for a month. Give yourself definite goals such as these and see if you can attain them on a regular basis.

Swami Sivananda advocates, with deep conviction, the necessity for keeping a spiritual diary, comparing week on week, month on month, adjusting and adapting to new situations as they arise. He encourages us to understand that we are keeping the diary solely for our own benefit; to maintain integrity and honesty in keeping it; to accept our faults openly, and to endeavour to rectify them in the future. He says: "Your diary is your guide and eye-opener. Through it you will get solace, peace of mind and contentment, you will understand the value of time and how it slips away. Start keeping a spiritual diary from this very moment and benefit from the marvellous results."

We urge you to start one today!

THE SPIRITUAL DIARY

We offer here a few pointers to creating a diary, which you can use as a guide. The sample chart below right provides a way of systematically recording and checking your progress.

Sleep
Record the time you went to bed and got up in the morning. How well did you sleep? Try to make your retiring and rising times regular. Avoid going to bed late and try to get up early, following nature's patterns. Too much sleep creates lethargy, too little weakens the brain.

Asanas and pranayama
Record how long you spent in asanas and pranayama, two simple and supreme ways of maintaining good health.

Meditation
For how long did you meditate? Thirty minutes twice a day is what you should aim for. If you can't manage this, thirty minutes once a day will be highly beneficial. Be regular in your practice, trying not to miss even one day.

Karma yoga

Try to work without expectations of reward, and with love and respect for the work, whatever it is you are doing. Record your daily success in karma yoga.

Charity

If you can, give a little to charity each week. As well as money, try to give goods or time. As you practice generosity, your heart will open.

Physical exercise

Record your progress with a routine of exercising for half an hour a day to keep you fit in both mind and body.

Diet

Keep to a healthy diet and make a note of where you failed: what you ate, drank, or smoked to break your resolve. Following the simple dietary suggestions in this book will increase your willpower as well as your health.

Personal conduct

Ask yourself what lies you told, of whom you were jealous, how much you worried, and how many times you were angry. Try to pinpoint one or two character defects and work with them in a gentle but disciplined manner. Using techniques outlined in Chapter Four, start to whittle away at fear, which manifests as worry and anxiety, and anger, which manifests as irritability and impatience.

	MONDAY	TUESDAY	WEDNESDAY	THURSDAY	FRIDAY	SATURDAY	SUNDAY	AVERAGE OR TOTAL
Time to bed								
Time got up								
How many hours slept								
How many minutes spent in asanas								
How many minutes spent in pranayama								
How many minutes spent in meditation								
How many minutes spent in exercise								
How many minutes spent in karma yoga								
Charity gifts or work								
How many instances of lying or anger								
How many instances of worry or anxiety								
How many instances of kindness or generosity								

CHOOSING A SPIRITUAL GUIDE

*Do not dig many wells or shallow pits
here and there for getting water.
Dig a deep pit in one place...
Drink deep from one well...
Following many people or spiritual paths
will land you in confusion and dilemma.
One will tell you to do one thing
and another something else.
Listen to all but follow one.
Respect all but adore one.*

SWAMI SIVANANDA

We know that when we want to acquire new knowledge, we need guidance. In our work, sports and leisure activities, and in our emotional lives we turn to those who can help us. Friends, family, and colleagues as well as professionals act as guides on the path to newly acquired knowledge: we trust that this guidance, based on their experience, is necessary and valid and we don't question it.

In the same way, when we want to go deeper into our spiritual practice, a teacher or guide is essential to help us overcome some of the challenges and obstacles that crop up as we evolve (see Chapter Ten). Swami Sivananda gives a beautiful analogy of how spiritual knowledge is passed on from the teacher to the student. He says that to light a candle, you need a candle already alight. Similarly, an enlightened soul alone can give light to another soul.

As our practice unfolds, we have to deal with emotions and thoughts that we may not have experienced before and we may not know how to handle them. Questions may arise and will remain unanswered if there is no one to advise us. We may give up our practice if we cannot clear our doubts. Or we may lose sight of our goal and get sidetracked by the continual distractions of life, or be overwhelmed by our shortcomings or the apparent lack of improvement in our mental state. Spiritual life is beset with challenges, known only to those who have patiently trodden the way for many years and worked hard to unravel the complexities of the mind. The path of meditation can be compared to a long journey where roadmaps are not readily available and the road signs unclear. Anyone who goes deeper into a spiritual practice finds that they cannot rely on intellect and willpower alone. The ego will tell us that we can do it alone, that we don't need help, that we are clever enough to find our own way. It may even fool us into believing that we are already quite advanced on the path, a path often likened to a razor's edge, when the truth is that we have hardly begun. For this reason we need someone to guide us.

Your teacher will guide you on your path and will warn you of the challenges. He or she will adjust your practice when necessary. He will act as a mirror and help you to see the limitations of your ego-consciousness, a painful but necessary process. This is not something you can do alone. Just as you cannot see your own back, so also you cannot see your own misconceptions and shortcomings. The ego greatly dislikes them being pointed out. Nevertheless, no real progress can be made without letting go of the ego-consciousness.

Even if you have a teacher, it is important to continue studying on your own. Reading spiritual books is an enriching and inspiring discipline and offers a framework for further practice (hence this book). But classical spiritual scriptures are likened to a forest, dense and tricky to navigate. Many of the writings are ambiguous

and contain contradictory passages full of esoteric meanings, cross-references, and hidden explanations. We need instruction to unravel their mysteries. Even simpler books, however well written, cannot replace the watchful eye of an experienced teacher.

Some great masters are able to reach the goal without the help of a teacher, but this happens rarely and we should not assume we have reached such a level of evolution. For some, it is also possible to choose someone who is no longer physically present as a spiritual teacher. Ultimately, the real teacher is within your heart and guidance from within is the highest form of learning. Creating a connection with the Divine is not instantaneous; it takes perseverance and patience to develop the sincere devotion necessary for direct guidance. Nevertheless, it will come if you are earnest and sincere in your practice.

How to find a teacher

If you find peace in the presence of a person, if you are inspired by his words, if he can clear your doubts, then you can take him as your spiritual teacher. Other qualities to look for in a teacher are selflessness, detachment, compassion, humility, and an absence of greed, anger, and lust. If possible, the student should live for a time in same environment as the teacher, which is the traditional way of receiving spiritual knowledge. Sometimes it is not easy to find such a very evolved teacher. In this case, look for one who has been treading the path for some time and has achieved a certain level of evolution and mastery in yoga and meditation, and who follows the teaching of a self-realized master. Meditation on a picture of such a realized master will bring you inspiration and uplift your mind. If you sincerely want spiritual guidance, it will come to you, sometimes in an unexpected way – your teacher may even appear in your dreams. The difficulty is not usually in finding the teacher, but lies more in the readiness of the student to learn, as the story below illustrates.

Once upon a time a student came to learn from a master. The master with his insight was able to see that the student's mind was not quite ready to learn, being full of egoism, vanity, and ignorance. The master offered to pour a cup of tea for the student. He kept pouring and pouring until the tea spilled over the cup. Annoyed and surprised, the student shouted out: "You are spilling the tea all over my hand!" Then the master said: "This cup is just like your mind, already full. Empty the cup of your mind, so that knowledge may be poured into it."

In ancient times, students approached their teachers with great humility and patience. Nowadays, we tend to seek instant results. We want quick changes, a magical pill for instant meditation. Nature teaches us that every process of growth takes time and requires tremendous patience. There are no short cuts in spiritual life.

The relationship between a teacher and a student is based on loving respect and spiritual understanding. It is intimate and sacred. You want to open your heart to your teacher and this capacity to trust and open up will speed up your spiritual progress a great deal. The role of the teacher is to give guidance, encouragement, and loving support. However, he cannot do the work for you. The work of uplifting the mind is yours alone.

CHAPTER TEN

CHALLENGES TO MEDITATION

You will find meditation much easier if you have a comprehensive understanding of the challenges that may arise during your practice. In this chapter we will look at a few of these and offer guidance on how to deal with them.

By now you will know that the practice of meditation asks for close introspection that leads to changes in personality, lifestyle, and values. You will have discovered that improving your way of life, strengthening your character, and dissolving shortcomings play an important part in bringing calmness and peacefulness to the mind, which is in turn a necessary condition for successful meditation. The work of changing behaviour and personality may be difficult, but see each hurdle as a test to strengthen the mind. The mind increases in power when it overcomes problematic situations.

When you begin to practise, it is common for layer upon layer of negative thoughts to come up from the subconscious as soon as you sit for meditation. Do not drive these thoughts out forcibly or suddenly, or they will turn against you with increased energy. Negative thoughts flood in if you try to get rid of them. This is a psychological law known as the Law of Resistance. Let them gently go and return to your mantra. You will know that your mind is strengthening when you feel uneasy as negative thoughts arise; previously these thoughts would have been welcomed. Keep on watching the mind, particularly when it is relaxed. Waves of anger, irritability, jealousy, and hatred are the enemies of meditation, peace, and wisdom. Chapter Three offers advice on how to rid yourself of these thoughts effectively.

SLEEP

Drowsiness and sleep are common obstacles in the practice of meditation. The amount of sleep you need will be reduced quite considerably once you establish a regular practice. Yoga considers

the need for sleep to be psychological and teaches that it is possible to slowly reduce the hours you sleep each night. Through your yogic practices you develop a calm and steady mind, become more relaxed, and consequently require less sleep.

Sometimes during your practice you may be unsure whether you have slipped into sleep or whether you are still actually meditating. During meditation the body is light and the mind is cheerful, but during sleep the body and eyelids are heavy and the mind is dull. If sleep becomes a problem during meditation, splash cold water on your face, do breathing exercises, or stand on your head for five minutes (see page 44) and you will revive.

LETHARGY

Lethargy and depression often affect the beginner in meditation. Sometimes the cause is physical, such as poor eating habits, indigestion, lack of exercise, or a disruptive environment. Take care of your health and wellbeing with regular exercise and a healthy diet, and by avoiding tedious mental work, too much or too little sleep, and excessive sexual activity. Lethargy can also set in when life is unbalanced. Bring a rhythm into your life, by establishing a daily routine of meditation, exercise, and study. Give some time to charity. These practices enliven the mind and lessen the tendency to slip back into inertia. Physical activity provides the necessary balance for the practice of meditation, and hard work should become an integral part of each day's structure. Because body and mind are intimately connected, try to be cheerful at all times. Cheerfulness and good health walk hand in hand.

TOO MUCH TALKING

Excessive talking diminishes spiritual power and hinders the practice of meditation. Talking requires a considerable amount of energy and makes a person restless and agitated. If you are a talkative person or if you enjoy intellectual debate, beware of the tendency to

engage in unnecessary chatter or discussions, which will leave you feeling drained. The wise speak few words and only when necessary.

To help calm, centre, and discipline the mind, try to practice *mouna*, silence, for up to an hour every day, over and above the time spent in meditation. For maximum effect, practise at a time when there is usually a great temptation to talk. Obviously, the idea is not to seem surly and unfriendly or to cause bad feeling. Practise with sensitivity. Resisting the temptation to engage in conversation or discussion at every opportunity can be regarded as a form of mouna. It will strengthen your willpower and conserve your energy.

If you are withdrawn or shy, do not use the practice of mouna as a means to maintain your isolation. Mouna is used solely for the purpose of channelling the energy dissipated in talking to a higher practice, such as japa, prayer, or *svadhyaya*, the study of spiritual writings (see pages 118–19).

Self-justification along with the traits of self-assertion, obstinacy, dissimulation, and lying are associated with talking too much. One lie follows another in a succession of attempts at self-justification. If you can readily admit faults, mistakes, and weaknesses, your mind will start to calm and meditation becomes easier.

NEGATIVE INFLUENCES

Negative influences include anybody or anything that pulls the mind away from peacefulness. Try to protect yourself carefully from influences that may draw you into negativity and, if at all possible, avoid people who lie or steal, or are greedy, or indulge in criticism and gossip. Unfavourable surroundings, books and music that create discontent, all distract the mind, draw it outwards rather than allow it to focus inwards, and fill it with desires it would not normally have. Try to associate only with those whose aspirations are uplifting and inspiring.

DISCOURAGEMENT

After a while, doubts may arise about the effectiveness of practising meditation. Lack of faith is discouraging and a serious obstacle in the path of personal development. You may be tempted to reduce your efforts or even give up altogether. Remember that there will always be periods when progress seems a little slow. Doubt has the tendency to appear again and again. Whenever it arises, immediately seek out inspiring friends or teachers and stay with them for a while. Conversing with people of strong faith and firm practice clears all doubts. Right inquiry and reasoning can be supported by the study of uplifting books. Let go of confusion by the courage of conviction and by faith based on reason. Keep reminding yourself that challenges help to strengthen you. Continue the practice, with no regard for the outcome. Growth comes, but it is always gradual. Sincerity, regularity, and patience will bring progress.

ANGER

Of all the emotional barriers to the practice of meditation, one of the most devastating is anger, the greatest enemy of peace. When desires are not gratified, anger manifests. Your mind becomes confused, memory and understanding are lost; you say and do things with a lack of awareness and control. Anger does great damage to our physical and psychic bodies, as well as to those of others. The whole nervous system can be shattered by one angry outburst. Anger gains strength with repetition and is difficult to control once it becomes habitual.

When you control anger, all other shortcomings die by themselves and the will gradually strengthens. Watch your mind carefully for signs of irritability. If you get irritated frequently, try strengthening the mind by practising patience as soon as irritation manifests. This way you will be able to stop the impulses and emotions before they take form and escape out of control. Always speak moderately, and if you feel anger rising during conversation, stop speaking and turn

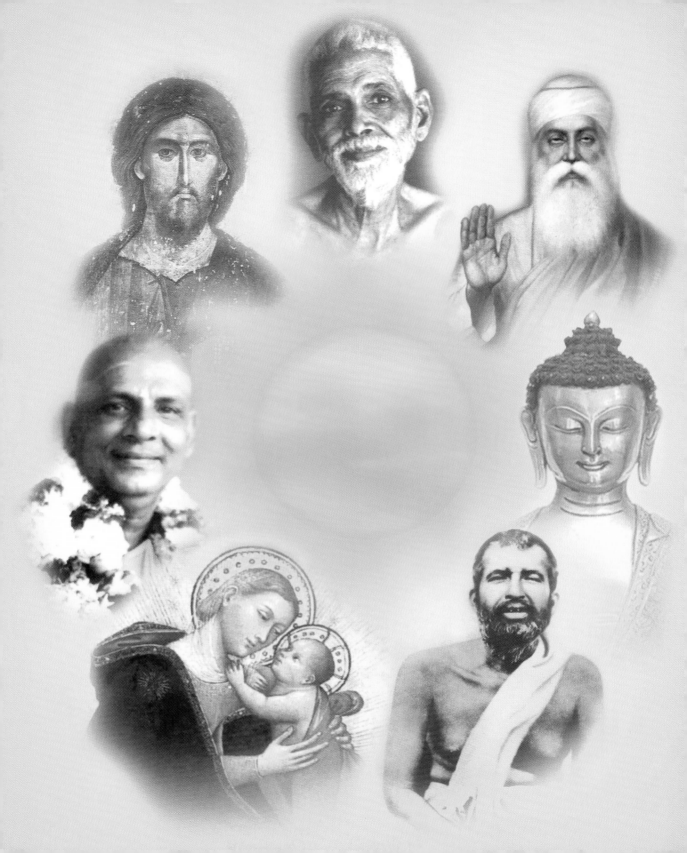

your attention elsewhere. Drinking cool water or taking a brisk walk will also help. Try to speak authoritatively but gently, as harsh words only create upset. Smoking, eating meat, and drinking alcohol have the effect of increasing rajas (see page 36), which aggravates the mind. They are best avoided.

FEAR

Fear is the most debilitating of all emotions and will severely hamper your ability to meditate. Constant fear, of which worry and anxiety are expressions, saps your energy, shakes your confidence, and undermines your ability to succeed. Fear is a result of a lively imagination, but nonetheless assumes real forms and manifests in a variety of ways: fear of death, fear of disease, fear of solitude, fear of company. Fear of public criticism especially can stand in the way of your meditation progress. Friends, colleagues, and even close family may mock or criticize you for your practice. Hold on to your practice, even in the face of ridicule.

HATRED

Hatred, like anger and fear, is one of the greatest obstacles to the mind of the serious practitioner. Hatred is like a contagious disease. Hatred creates more hatred, resulting ultimately in the horror and devastation of war. Its roots are often deeply embedded in the subconscious mind. Contempt, prejudice, and ridicule are some of the most damaging of the many forms that hatred takes. Conflicts such as those between Catholics and Protestants, and Jews and Muslims show how prejudice can lead to centuries of discord and suffering. You can have your own principles and your own standards and modes of behaviour and still respect the viewpoints and actions of others. Truth is not the sole monopoly of any one person, group, or spiritual system.

Meditate on saints, sages, and divine incarnations. Clockwise from top left: Christ, Ramana Maharshi, Guru Nanak, Buddha, Rama Krishna Paramahamsa, Mary and the child Jesus, Swami Sivananda

Gossip, criticizing, and judging are some of the more subtle manifestations of hatred. Finding fault in other people and busying oneself with someone else's affairs are destructive habits that create restlessness and agitation in the mind. Peace of mind and universal peace are possible only when hatred, prejudice, and bigotry have been replaced with love.

DWELLING IN THE PAST

When you sit for meditation, vivid thoughts of past experiences may appear. You may remember events that have been buried in your subconscious for many years. Memories of conversations or lost loved ones will agitate the mind and make the practice of meditation difficult. The imagination can play havoc with the past, creating imbalance and disharmony in the mind. As you get older there is a tendency for the mind to dwell more frequently in the events of long ago, preventing you from living life fully in the present. Dreams of childhood, schooldays, and youth are just dreams and should be laid gently and permanently to rest. Try to let go of all thoughts of the past, both distant and recent, and live fully in the present.

THE EGO

The ego behind the mask of the human personality is one of the biggest hurdles to overcome in order to achieve lasting peace. For Westerners who are taught to revere individuality, the need to surrender the ego is especially difficult to understand. The ego is the sense of "I-ness" or "my-ness", which manifests as selfishness and a feeling of separation from the world. Overconfident people are usually considered to have a big ego, but people who are very shy and withdrawn also possess a large ego; their sense of me, my, and mine is equally strong.

The ego loves its own ideas and impulses, and balks at change. Dissimulation, hypocrisy, exaggeration, and secretiveness are traits of a dominant ego. A powerful ego clouds the intellect. You may lie

in order to cover up your mistakes, to maintain your position, to pander to your own ideas, or to indulge in bad habits. You may use self-justification, or deny faults and defects, and you may be totally unaware of the consequences of actions propelled by your selfish desire. Often those with inflated egos do not know what they mean, and do not mean what they say; they become too self-willed and self-satisfied to see clearly what is happening in their minds.

Try to introspect and accept your shortcomings. Be easy on yourself and have compassion when you discover aspects of your personality that your ego would rather not see. You cannot expect perfection at this stage, and if you can accept errors and mistakes in your character you have won half the battle. Change will come once acceptance is there. With regular meditation and strong determination to eradicate egoism, you will develop a powerful and selfless will. Then with persistent and dedicated work, you will start to see positive changes in your personality and behaviour.

CHAPTER ELEVEN

AS THE PRACTICE DEEPENS

Spiritual practices can often be confused with psychic experiences. In this chapter we outline briefly some of the psychic phenomena that may arise during your meditation practice. Experiencing them can feel at the least out of the ordinary and at the most quite alarming. We include them, as a book on meditation would not be complete without them. But the yoga masters warn us that they are not the goal of meditation, that we may never experience them, and that if we do we should not get sidetracked by them. They are only a natural occurrence and are to be treated as such, as signs that the mind and consciousness are simply expanding.

As your practice deepens, guard against a feeling of moral superiority towards those who are not on the same path. Spiritual arrogance and self-satisfaction are more insidious forms of the arrogance encountered in daily living. Spiritual hypocrisy, a related weakness, may also emerge in those who have made some progress but have not yet thoroughly mastered their shortcomings. You may pretend to be what you are not, making an elaborate outward show of your apparent spirituality. For those travelling the spiritual path, there is no greater error than using spirituality to take advantage of trusting people. The masters say that spiritual hypocrisy is much worse than ordinary hypocrisy, as it makes a mockery of timeless wisdom. They urge us to be constantly on the alert for tendencies towards any form of spiritual egoism and to see ourselves merely as instruments of the Absolute. We need to increase our efforts to practise humility through selfless service, and to deepen our devotion to our goal, our teacher, and the Absolute.

LIGHT

Different lights can appear in the mind during meditation. Bright white lights or lights of many colours including yellow, red, blue, green, and purple can manifest. There may be small balls of floating light, a full blaze, or flashes like lightning, fire, burning charcoal, fire-

flies, the sun, the moon, and the stars. All these demonstrate that the mind is steadying and concentration is deepening. At first, these lights are irregular; they appear and then immediately fade, causing sensations of extreme joy and happiness. With time they remain for up to thirty minutes depending on the strength and degree of your concentration. Try to keep a steady posture and breathe slowly. Sometimes the light is so powerful that you need to break the meditation. But with constant practice, the phenomenon will become familiar and any fears you may have will disappear.

INNER SOUNDS

Anahata sounds are the mystic inner sounds heard during deep meditation. Hearing them is a sign of the purification of the *nadis* or psychic nerve channels, due to the sustained practice of pranayama. You may hear the musical sounds of a bell, flute, or kettle drum, the sound of a conch shell being blown, or the natural sounds of thunder or the humming of a bee. Anahata sounds are heard through the right ear and are most distinct when both ears are held closed. To do this, sit cross-legged, blocking the ears with the right and left thumbs, the eyes with the forefingers, and the nostrils with the middle fingers. Then pinch the mouth shut with the ring and little fingers. This hand position is called the *yoni mudra* (see left). Listen very attentively to hear the mystic sounds, which are vibrations of prana in the heart.

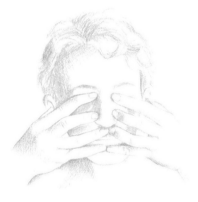

The yoni mudra, in which the thumb and fingers block the ears, eyes, nose, and mouth.

VISIONS OF THE ASTRAL PLANE

You may have visions that belong to the astral plane – of gods, celestial maidens, angels, beautiful flower gardens, palatial buildings, rivers, mountains, and golden temples. Sometimes you may see elementals, strange looking astral creatures that appear simply as a test of courage. Beings living in the astral plane are similar to those of the physical world but without a physical overcoat. They have desires and cravings just as humans have. They have subtle bodies with powers of materialization and dematerialization and they can move about freely. They come down to encourage or test you.

HOLY VISIONS

Your *ishta devata*, that aspect of the Absolute to whom you are devoted, may appear to you in your meditation practice. You will feel light, bliss, knowledge, and divine love flowing from this presence to you. You may have conversations with Him or Her. However, once you attain cosmic consciousness, these conversations will stop. You will savour the language of silence, the language of the heart.

ASTRAL TRAVEL

During the course of your practice, you may experience the feeling of separation from your body. This experience brings joy mixed with anxiety; joy at the possession of a new, light, astral body; anxiety at being on an unknown plane. Initially, your consciousness feels undeveloped, like that of a newborn puppy with just-opened eyes. You may have the sensation of rotating or floating in an atmosphere filled with golden lights, objects, and beings. When you return to your physical body, it feels as though you are gliding smoothly back into it through a fine tube-like opening.

After experiencing this, you will clearly understand the difference between life in the physical and astral planes. You will have an intense desire to return and remain in that state of consciousness. In the beginning, you will not be able to sustain your stay in the astral plane for longer than a few minutes. But if you continue your practice with patience, perseverance, and firmness, you will be able to leave your body at will and stay in the astral plane for longer. Once you can remain there for two or three hours, you will be free from identifying with your body. This means that you will understand that you are not your body, that you have an existence outside the physical plane.

Contemplating the beauty of the physical world helps to expand our mind and make us aware of the existence of higher planes of consciousness.

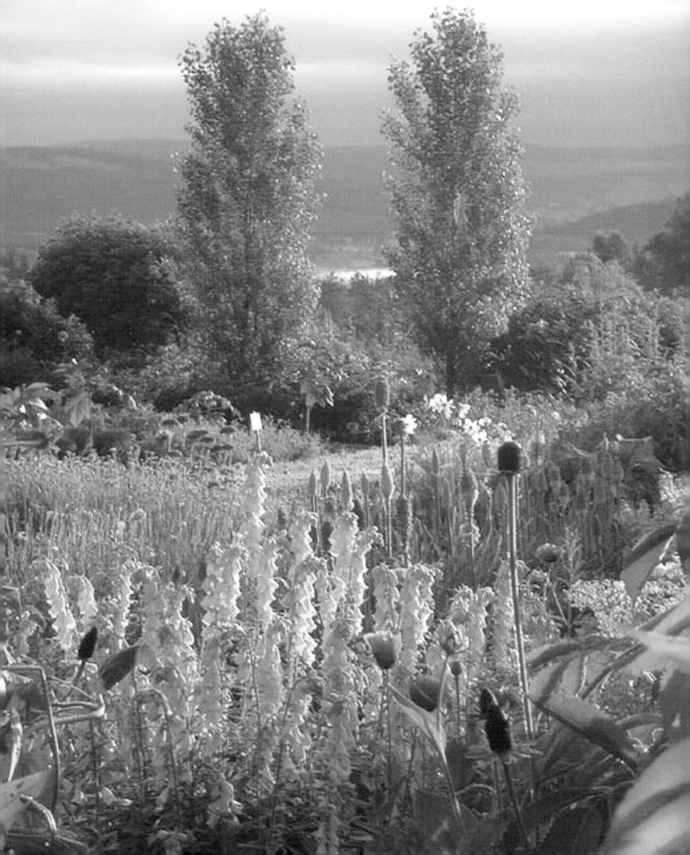

CHAPTER TWELVE

THE EXPANDED VISION

Once the mind is purified and free from imbalances, deep meditation becomes possible. In this state, you do not perceive the object on which you are concentrating as separate from yourself. You perceive it as pure thought vibration. If you focus on a mantra, for instance, there will be no more awareness of its meaning, no perception of its gross sound. As you identify with the object of your concentration, giving it your full attention, you perceive it from within and automatically receive knowledge of the object. Here you enter a subtle state of transcendental bliss in which a sense of duality remains: you are still aware of subject (you) and object (the object of concentration).

Once you have sustained this state of meditation for some time, you will enter the state of *samadhi* or cosmic consciousness, a state of bliss in which the subject, the object and the mental connection between the two become one. The senses, the intellect, and the emotions are transcended and you obtain complete identification with, or absorption into, the object of concentration. Even pure thought is transcended, as you merge with the object of your focus and all that remains is the experience of everything dissolving into one consciousness.

Samadhi is not an imaginary experience or a hypnotic trance, but occurs when the third eye or the eye of wisdom opens. The result is a complete annihilation of greed and egoism, experienced as a state of peace and joy that cannot be described in words. Samadhi is the ultimate goal of the entire practice of meditation and yoga.

Experiencing samadhi will bring about a complete transformation in your personality: you will know true spiritual relaxation and feel the release of a great amount of spiritual energy. You will receive inspiration, grace, and spiritual strength. You will be aware of the unity of all things. You will be aware of the purpose of your life. You will develop a keen desire and willingness to engage in selfless

Mount Kailas in Tibet is sacred to both Buddhists and Hindus and is the eternal abode of Lord Siva.

Feel the silence
Hear the silence
Taste the silence
Silence is the music of your soul

SWAMI VISHNU-DEVANANDA

service. You will be free from fear of death. You will move away from the sense of ego and see the Self in all beings and all beings in the Self. Ultimately, the goal of the experienced yogi is to be able to maintain this state at all times. It will become his or her natural state, so that life becomes one unbroken meditation. This is the advanced state that yoga calls self-realization.

As beginners on the path, our challenge is to keep alive our aspiration to expand our consciousness. The mind tends always to slip back into its small ways.

A journey of a thousand miles starts with a single step. Take this first step on the road of spiritual knowledge by beginning your meditation practice now. There is nothing in the world that matches the depth of knowledge and wisdom that is offered by meditation. Happiness cannot come from power, wealth, and fame – deep abiding peace comes only from the realization that we are all one, and meditation is the supreme instrument to take us there.

Let us conclude with the words of a self-realized teacher, Swami Sivananda, describing this consciousness of the unity of all things:

See life as a whole. The world is one home.
All are members of one human family.
No one is independent of that whole.
We make ourselves miserable by separating from others.
Separation means death. Cultivate cosmic love.
Include all.
Destroy all barriers that separate one human being
from another. Protect life. Protect animals.
Let all life be sacred.
Then this world will be a haven of peace.
Smile with the flowers, play with the butterflies and birds.
Talk to the rainbow, the wind, the stars and the sun.
Develop friendship with your neighbours,
dogs, cats, trees, and flowers.
You will have a wide, rich and full life.
You will realize the full unity of life.

SWAMI SIVANANDA

GLOSSARY

A

Agni sara – the power or essence of fire; one of the six classical kriyas (purification techniques)

Ahimsa – first of the five yamas (restraints); non-violence

Ajna chakra – sixth psychic centre situated between the eyebrows

Anahata chakra – fourth psychic centre situated in the heart area

Anahata sounds – mystical sounds heard in meditation

Ananda – spiritual bliss

Anuloma viloma – alternate-nostril breathing exercise, a pranayama

Aparigraha – one of the five yamas (restraints); non-covetousness

Arati – a devotional practice in which light is offered in front of a sacred space (altar, holy river, etc.)

Asana – literally seat; posture (the third step of raja yoga)

Ashram – a hermitage; a place, usually in nature, where students and teachers live and practise yoga

Asteya – one of the five yamas (restraints); non-stealing

Astral body – a subtle body; the "body of light"; a body of the mind and the senses, out of which proceeds the gross body of matter, to which it is connected by an astral cord

Astral plane – a subtle plane

Astral travel – a temporary separation of the astral body from the physical body, which occurs in dream sleep or during meditation or other spiritual experiences

Avatar – literally one who descends; an incarnation of God

Ayurveda – literally science or knowledge of life; traditional Indian medicine

B

Bhagavad Gita – literally Song of God; one of the most important scriptures of yoga

Bhakti yoga – the path of devotion in yoga

Brahmacharya – one of the five yamas (restraints); control of the senses and more specifically, celibacy

Brahmamuhurta – the period of an hour and a half before sunrise, which is the most conducive for the practice of meditation

Brahman – the Godhead, the Absolute

C

Chakra – literally a wheel; a psychic centre located in the astral body

Chin mudra – a hand position in which the thumb and index finger touch lightly. The gesture symbolizes spiritual knowledge

D

Devata – a deity; divine power

Devavani – literally the language of gods; another name for the Sanskrit language

Dharana – concentration (the sixth step of raja yoga); from the Sanskrit root *dhr* to hold firmly, to fix

Dharma – righteous conduct; universal law

Dhyana – meditation (the seventh step of raja yoga)

E

Ekagrata – one-pointed

Elemental – a being that lives on the astral plane

G

Gunas – qualities of nature

H

Hatha – *ha* (sun), *tha* (moon); a system of yoga that focuses on controlling and harmonizing the subtle energies of the body

I

Ishta devata – a particular form of God that one is devoted to

Ishvara – God as perceived through the manifested universe (as opposed to God as absolute consciousness)

Ishvara prandihana – one of the five niyamas (observances); devotion or surrender to God

J

Japa – repetition of a mantra

Japa mala – a string of beads used in the practice of japa

Jnana yoga – the path of knowledge

K

Kapalabhati – pumping breath, an exercise that is both a kriya (cleansing technique) and a pranayama

Karma – an action; the Law of Karma – the law of action and reaction

Karma yoga – the path of selfless service

Kriya – a cleansing technique

Kshipta - literally thrown or scattered; a distracted state of the mind

Kundalini energy – primordial cosmic energy in the individual

Kundalini yoga – a branch of raja yoga whose aim is to awaken the kundalini energy

L

Laya chintana – literally absorption; concentration on the mind with a view to dissolving it back into its original cause

Likhita japa – mantra writing

M

Maha mantra – literally great mantra

Mala – rosary

Manasika japa – mental repetition of a mantra

Mantra – a mystical energy encased in a sound structure

Mantra shakti – the inherent energy of a mantra

Meru – the central and usually the largest bead in a mala (rosary)

Mouna – observance of silence

Mudha – a dull state of the mind

N

Nadis – subtle energy channels in the astral body

Neti-neti – literally not-this, not-this; a vedantic technique for meditation

Nirguna – without qualities

Niruddha – literally suspended; a state of mind in which all thought waves are controlled

Niyamas – a set of five ethical observances (the second step in raja yoga)

O

Ojas – spiritual energy; the essence of all seven dhatus (tissues) in the body

OM – the sacred syllable symbolizing the Absolute, Brahman

P

Padmasana – the lotus position

Parigraha – hoarding wealth or possessions

Patanjali – a great sage who compiled the *Raja Yoga Sutras*, one of the most important texts on yoga

Prana – vital energy

Pranayama – the control of prana, vital energy (the fourth step of raja yoga)

Pratyahara – withdrawal of the senses (the fifth step of raja yoga)

R

Raja yoga – the eight-step path of yoga based on meditation

Rajas – one of three qualities or gunas; the principle of activity

Rishi – a seer of Truth

S

Sabdabrahman – sound-form of Brahman, the causal vibration of the universe

Sadhana shakti – energy activated by spiritual practice (sadhana)

Saguna – with a form

Sahasrara chakra – the seventh chakra in the astral body, located at the top of the head

Sakshi aham - literally "I am Witness"

Sakshi bhav – an attitude of detached witnessing of one's own thoughts

Samadhi – the superconscious state experienced as bliss

Samskara – an impression; tendency

Sannyasin – a monk or nun; one who has embraced a life of complete renunciation

Sanskrit – "the language of the gods"; it is considered to be the one of the oldest languages in the world and is the language of the yoga scriptures

Santosha – one of the five niyamas (observances); contentment

Satsang – the company of wise or spiritually-minded people

Sattva – one of three qualities or gunas; the principle of purity and light

Satya – one of the five yamas (restraints); truth

Saucha – one of the five niyamas (observances); purity

Shakti – cosmic energy

Siddhasana – literally the adept's pose; one of the sitting positions used for meditation

Solar plexus – a main nerve network in the system located below the stomach; also the system's main energy centre

Steya – stealing, theft

Sukham sthiram – literally a comfortable and firm position; a description of the meditative pose from the *Raja Sutras*

Sutra – literally a thread; a verse, aphorism

Svadharma – personal duty (dharma)

Svadhyaya – one of five niyamas (observances); study of the scriptures; introspection

Swami – a monk or nun; literally owner, lord, leader

Swami Sivananda – one of the greatest modern sages of India; the inspiration behind the Sivananda Yoga Vedanta Centres; teacher of Swami Vishnu-devananda

Swami Vishnu-devananda – founder of the Sivananda Yoga Vedanta Centres; a world-renowned teacher and author of *Meditation and Mantras* and the best-seller *The Complete Illustrated Book of Yoga*

T

Tamas – one of three qualities or gunas; the principle of inertia, dullness, darkness

Tapas – literally fire; one of the five niyamas (observances); austerity

Tratak – gazing; a kriya (cleansing technique) and a concentration exercise

U

Upamsu japa – whispering of a mantra

Upanishads – the revealed scriptures of the *Vedas* containing the essence of the philosophy of vedanta

V

Vaikhari japa – audible repetition of a mantra

Varna – a colour

Vedanta – literally the end of the *Vedas*; the highest philosophy based on the *Upanishads*

Vedas – the most ancient of the scriptures in India

Vikshipta – a state of partial concentration of the mind

Vritti – a thought wave

Y

Yamas – ethical restraints (the first step of raja yoga)

Yoga – literally union; union of the individual soul with the Supreme Soul; a system of spiritual disciplines that aims at such a union

Yoga Sutras – aphorisms on yoga compiled by the sage Patanjali

Yogi – one who practises or has achieved yoga

Yoni mudra – a hand position that creates a specific energy pattern conducive to concentration of the mind

KEY TO SANSKRIT TRANSLITERATION

अ	*a*	but	ग	*ga*	go	ध	*dha*	redhead
आ	*ā*	father	घ	*gha*	log hut	न	*na*	name
इ	*i*	it	ङ	*ṅ*	sing	प	*pa*	pot
ई	*ī*	beet	च	*ca*	chunk	फ	*pha*	loophole
उ	*u*	put	छ	*cha*	church-hall	ब	*ba*	basket
ऊ	*ū*	pool	ज	*ja*	Jeremy	भ	*bha*	abhor
ऋ	*ṛ*	rhythm	झ	*jha*	hedgehog	म	*ma*	music
ॠ	*ṝ*	reed	ञ	*ñ*	enjoy	य	*ya*	you
ऌ	*ḷ*	jewelry	ट	*ṭa*	start	र	*ra*	drama
ए	*e*	play	ठ	*ṭha*	anthill	ल	*la*	lime
ऐ	*ai*	high	ड	*ḍa*	dark	व	*va*	van
ओ	*o*	toe	ढ	*ḍha*	godhead	श	*śa*	shine
औ	*au*	loud	ण	*ṇa*	bundle	ष	*ṣa*	efficient
क	*ka*	skate	त	*ta*	street	स	*sa*	serve
ख	*kha*	black hat	थ	*tha*	table	ह	*ha*	hat
			द	*da*	do			

ABOUT THE SIVANANDA YOGA VEDANTA CENTRES

The Sivananda Yoga Vedanta Centres dedicate themselves to promoting the yogic lifestyle, based on the five points laid down by Swami Vishnu-devananda:

1. Proper exercise
2. Proper breathing
3. Proper relaxation
4. Proper diet
5. Positive thinking
   and meditation.

The centres and ashrams are organized as spiritual communities, in each of which a group of people live and teach the yogic life. They practise daily meditation, asanas (yoga postures), and pranayama (breathing techniques), have a vegetarian diet, follow the ethical principles of yoga, and serve the community by teaching this lifestyle to people of all faiths and backgrounds.

ASHRAMS

Sivananda Yoga Retreat House
Am Bichlag Weg 40A
A6370 Reith bei Kitzbühel
Austria
Tel +43.5356.67.404
Fax +43.5356.67.404.4
e-mail tyrol@sivananda.org

Sivananda Ashram Yoga Retreat
PO Box N7550
Paradise Island, Nassau
Bahamas
Tel +1.242.363.2902
Fax +1.242.363.3783
e-mail Nassau@sivananda.org

Sivananda Ashram Yoga Camp
673 Eighth Avenue
Val Morin, Quebec J0T 2R0
Canada
Tel +1.819.322.3226
Fax +1.819.322.5876
e-mail HQ@sivananda.org

Sivananda Yoga Château
26 Impasse du Bignon
45170 Neuville aux Bois
France
Tel +33.2.38.91.88.82
Fax +33.2.38.91.18.09
e-mail Orleans@sivananda.org

Sivananda Yoga Vedanta Dhanwantari
Ashram
PO Neyyar Dam
Thiruvananthapuram Dt
Kerala 695 576
India
Tel +91.471.2273.093
Fax +91.471.2272.093
e-mail YogaIndia@sivananda.org

Sivananda Kutir
PO Netala
Uttara Kashi Dt
(near Siror Bridge)
Uttaranchal, Himalayas, 249 193
India
Tel +91.1374.222624
Fax +91.1374.224159
e-mail sivanandakutir@rediffmail.com

Sivananda Ashram Yoga Farm
14651 Ballantree Lane, Comp. 8
Grass Valley, CA 95949
USA
Tel +1.530.272.9322
Fax +1.530.477.6054
e-mail YogaFarm@sivananda.org

Sivananda Ashram Yoga Ranch
PO Box 195 Budd Road
Woodbourne, NY 12788
USA
Tel +1.845.436.6492
Fax +1.845.434.1032
e-mail YogaRanch@sivananda.org

CENTRES

Centro Internacional de Yoga
Sivananda
Julian Alvarez 2201
CP 1425 Buenos Aires
Argentina
Tel +54.11.4827.9269 / 9566
Fax +54.11.4827.9512
e-mail BuenosAires@sivananda.org

Sivananda Yoga Vedanta Zentrum
Prinz Eugenstrasse 18
A-1040 Vienna
Austria
Tel +43.1.586.3453
Fax +43.1.587.1551
e-mail Vienna@sivananda.org

Sivananda Yoga Vedanta Centre
5178 St Lawrence Blvd
Montreal, Quebec
H2T 1R8
Canada
Tel +1.514.279.3545
Fax +1.514.279.3527
e-mail Montreal@sivananda.org

Sivananda Yoga Vedanta Centre
77 Harbord Street
Toronto, Ontario
M5S 1G4
Canada
Tel +1.416.966.9642
Fax +1.416.966.1378
e-mail Toronto@sivananda.org

Centre de Yoga Sivananda Vedanta
123 Boulevard Sébastopol
F-75002 Paris
France
Tel +33.1.40.26.77.49
Fax +33.1.42.33.51.97
e-mail Paris@sivananda.org

Sivananda Yoga Vedanta Zentrum
Steinheilstrasse 1
D-8033 Munich
Germany
Tel +49.89.52.44.76
Fax +49.89.52.91.28
e-mail Munich@sivananda.org

Sivananda Yoga Vedanta Zentrum
Schmiljanstrasse 24
D-12161 Berlin
Germany
Tel +49.30.8599.9799
Fax +49.30.8599.9797
e-mail Berlin@sivananda.org

Sivananda Yoga Vedanta Nataraja
Centre
A-41 Kailas Colony
New Delhi 110 048
India
Tel +91.11.2648.0869/ 2645.3962
e-mail Delhi@sivananda.org

Sivananda Yoga Vedanta Centre
A-9, 7th Main Rd
Thiruvalluvavar Nagar
Thiruvanmiyur
Chennai 600 0841
India
Tel +91.44.2451.1626
e-mail Madras@sivananda.org

Sivananda Yoga Vedanta Centre
37/1929, West Fort, Airport Road
Thiruvananthapuram
Kerala 695 023
India
Tel +91.471.2450.942
Fax +91.471.2451.776
e-mail Trivandrum@sivananda.org

Sivananda Yoga Vedanta Centre
6 Lateris St
Tel Aviv 64166
Israel
Tel +972.3.691.6793
Fax +972.3.696.3939
e-mail TelAviv@sivananda.org

Centro de Yoga Sivananda Vedanta
Calle Eraso 4
E-28028 Madrid
Spain
Tel +34.91.361.5150
Fax +34.91.361.5194
e-mail Madrid@sivananda.org

Centre de Yoga Sivananda Vedanta
1 Rue de Minoteries
CH-1205 Geneva
Switzerland
Tel +41.22.328.03.28
Fax +41.22.328.03.59
e-mail Geneva@sivananda.org

Association de Yoga Sivananda
Acevedo Diaz 1523
11200 Montevideo
Uruguay
Tel +598.2.401.09.29 / 401.66.85
Fax +598.2.400.73.88
e-mail Montevideo@sivananda.org

Sivananda Yoga Vedanta Centre
51 Felsham Road
London SW15 1AZ
UK
Tel +44.020 8780.0160
Fax +44.020 8246.6450
e-mail London@sivananda.org

Sivananda Yoga Vedanta Center
243 West 24th Street
New York
NY 10011
USA
Tel +1.212.255.4560
Fax +1.212.727.7392
e-mail NewYork@sivananda.org

Sivananda Yoga Vedanta Center
1200 Arguella Blvd
San Francisco
CA 94122
USA
Tel +1.415.681.2731
Fax +1.415.681.5162
e-mail SanFrancisco@sivananda.org

Sivananda Yoga Vedanta Center
1246 Bryn Mawr
Chicago
Illinois 60660
USA
Tel +1.773.878.7771
Fax +1.773.878.7527
e-mail Chicago@sivananda.org

Sivananda Yoga Vedanta Center
Los Angeles
USA
Tel +1.310.822.9642/985.1022
e-mail LosAngeles@sivananda.org

BIOGRAPHIES

SWAMI SIVANANDA

Swami Sivananda was born into a devout Brahmin family in South India on 8 September 1887. He was a lively child, who even at an early age showed signs of great compassion. He had serious misgivings about the caste system, which was strictly upheld at the time, and as an adolescent he defied convention by taking fencing lessons from an "untouchable", an action quite unthinkable. He excelled at school and became a medical doctor at the age of twenty-three. In 1913 he travelled to Malaysia where he ran two hospitals connected to the rubber plantations and manned by thousands of Indian workers.

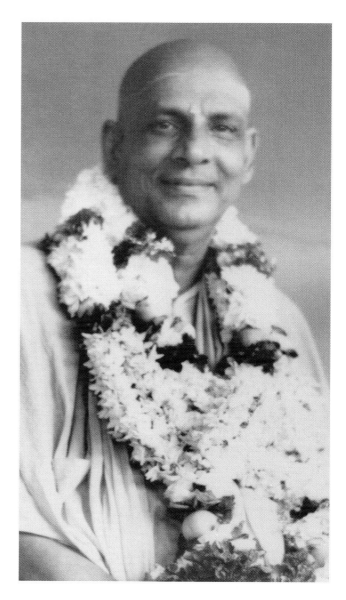

After ten years of dedicated service to the sick and poor, he left both Malaysia and his comfortable middle-class existence and became a wandering mendicant following the spiritual tradition of India. A year later he took holy orders and became a monk. His sincerity, his generosity, his humility, and his unalloyed compassion and joy drew around him many sincere men and women looking for guidance in lives beset with problems and pain. Swami Sivananda founded the Divine Life Society in 1939 and established his ashram on the banks of the holy River Ganges in Rishikesh, North India.

From then until his death, Swami Sivananda spent his time in teaching and serving in any way he was able. He was a prodigious writer – the author of over 200 books – and an inspiring and bold speaker. He was a giant of a man, physically, mentally, and spiritually, guiding many thousands the world over to live a rich and fulfilled life through the ancient teachings of yoga. His legacy is still felt strongly today through the flourishing Divine Life Society in Rishikesh and the many organizations that his disciples developed both in India and in the West. Swami Sivananda left his body on 14 July 1963. He is acknowledged as one of the great modern-day saints of India.

SWAMI VISHNU-DEVANANDA

In 1957 Swami Vishnu-devananda set out from the foothills of the Himalayas to carry out the bidding of his teacher Swami Sivananda. His instructions were to spread the teachings of yoga in the West. For thirty-seven years he worked tirelessly as a dedicated spiritual teacher, travelling around the world establishing centres and ashrams where this work could be accomplished.

Swami Vishnu-devananda was born Swamy Kuttan Nair on 31 December 1927 in the South Indian state of Kerala. After school he joined the Engineering Corps of the Indian Army. One day while on duty he found a pamphlet in a bin – its subject was the truth of spiritual practice and its author was Swami Sivananda. Swamy Kuttan Nair was so impressed that he took leave to visit Swami Sivananda, one of the great saints of modern times, in his ashram. After his discharge from the army, he became a schoolteacher for a short while, but in 1947 he left his life behind to follow his calling and enter the Sivananda Ashram in Rishikesh. Within a year, he had been ordained a monk and given the name Swami Vishnu-devananda.

He lived at the Sivananda Ashram for ten years, during which he was appointed as the first Professor of Hatha Yoga at the Yoga Vedanta Forest Academy. He also held a number of other positions, including that of personal secretary to Swami Sivananda.

He left India in 1957 and arrived on the West Coast of America, where it soon became apparent to him that people were so caught up in the whirlwind of their lives that they knew neither how to relax nor how to live healthily. Swami Vishnu-devananda devised the concept of the Yoga Vacation and set about creating places where people could have a complete rest of body, mind, and spirit. He founded several ashrams and centres based on an integrated approach to yoga. Used in the Sivananda Yoga

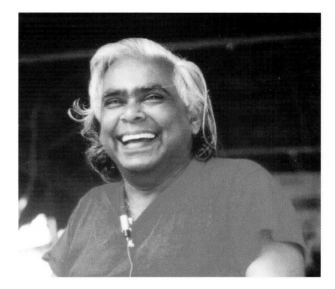

Centres today, this encompasses the four main paths of yoga, bhakti, jnana, raja, and karma, and the five points of yoga – proper exercise, proper breathing, proper relaxation, proper diet, and positive thinking and meditation.

In 1969 he founded the True World Order to create unity and understanding between the peoples of the world. He developed a unique Yoga Teachers' Training Course with the aim of bringing harmony in the world by teaching the basics of yoga discipline. In 1971 Swami Vishnu-devananda made headlines by flying around the world in his small two-seater plane dropping flowers and leaflets for peace over trouble-spots of the world. He sponsored numerous festivals, conferences, symposiums, and world tours – all calling for peace and understanding.

In addition to working tirelessly for world peace and being an inspiring teacher, Swami Vishnu-devananda is renowned for his books, *The Complete Illustrated Book of Yoga* and *Meditation and Mantras*. Swami Vishnu-devananda left his body on 9 November 1993, his legacy a worldwide organization dedicated to propagating the ancient and timeless wisdom of yoga.

INDEX

Figures in italics refer to illustrations

SUGGESTED READING

ACKNOWLEDGEMENTS

Books by Swami Sivananda
Published by the Divine Life Society,
Rishikesh 1998-2002

Bliss Divine

Commentary on the Bhagavad Gita

Concentration and Meditation

Conquest of Mind

Dhyana Yoga

*How to Cultivate Virtues and Eradicate
Vices*

Japa Yoga

*Life and Works of Swami Sivananda,
Volumes 1-5*

Mind Its Mysteries and Control

Raja Yoga

Sadhana

Science of Pranayama

*Sure Ways for Success in Life and God
Realization*

Books by Swami Vishnu-devananda

The Complete Illustrated Book of Yoga,
Three Rivers Press, 1998

Meditation and Mantras, Om Lotus
Publishing, 2000

*Commentary on the Hatha Yoga,
Pradipika*, Om Lotus Publishing, 1997

BOOKS BY THE SIVANANDA YOGA
VEDANTA CENTRE

The New Book of Yoga, Ebury Press,
2000

The Yoga Cookbook, Gaia Books, 1999

Yoga Mind and Body, Dorling
Kindersley, 1998

Learn Yoga in a Weekend, Dorling
Kindersley, 1996

101 Essential Tips of Yoga, Dorling
Kindersley, 1998

Further reading

Frawley, Dr David, *Ayurveda and the
Mind*, Lotus Press, 1996

Lad, Dr Vasant, *Ayurveda, the Science of
Self-Healing*, Lotus Press, 1985

Kisari Mohan Ganguli (commentary),
Bhagavad Gita, Munshiram Manoharlal
Publishers, 2002

Swami Venkatesananda, *The Concise
Yoga Vasishta*, SUNY, 1993

Swami Vivekananda, *Karma Yoga and
Bhakti Yoga*, Ramakrishna and
Vivekananda Center, 2000

Subramaniam, Kamal (retold by),
Mahabharata, Bharatiya Vidya Bhavan,
2000

Svoboda, Dr Robert, *Prakriti, Your
Ayurvedic Constitution*, Sadhana
Publications, 1998

Swami Vivekananda, *Raja Yoga*,
Ramakrishna and Vivekananda Center,
2000

Subramaniam, Kamal (retold by)
Ramayana, Bharatiya Vidya Bhavan,
1998

Subramaniam, Kamal (retold by) *Srimad
Bhagavatam*, Bharatiya Vidya Bhavan,
1997

Talks with Ramana Maharshi, Inner
Directions Publishing, 2001

Swami Venkatesananda (commentary),
Yoga Sutras of Patanjali, Divine Life
Society, 1998

Swami Nikhilananda (translation), *The
Gospel of Sri Ramakrishna*, Ramakrishna
and Vivekananda Center, 2000

Author's acknowledgements
The Sivananda Yoga Vedanta Centre
would like to thank Swami Kailasananda
(Florence Aillot) for writing the book
and Padmavati (Penny Collie) for her
editorial skills. We would also like to
thank the photographic models:
Swami Krishnapremananda (Emma
Brown), Narayan Chaitanya (Stefan
Barnert), Gopala (Darren Thomas),
and Savitri (Sarah Odell).

Publisher's acknowledgements
Gaia Books would like to thank Swami
Kailasananda for her patience, good
humour, and attention to detail in writing
the inspiring text she has produced with
Padmavati. Padmavati has worked
tirelessly as publishing liaison, and
facilitated the progress of the book
through all stages of production. We
thank all the members of the London
Centre and the members of Sivananda
Yoga Centres worldwide who have
helped with this project by supplying
photographs and other materials.
We thank particularly Swami
Krishnapremananda, Gopala, Savitri,
and Narayan Chaitanya, for their expert
skills in presenting the yoga poses for
photography.

Photo credits *by Permission of The
British Library Add.15297. folio. 93., 119;
Bruce Coleman Collection: 61 (apple tree)
Hans Reinhard, 62 Colin Varndell, 75
(acorn) Jane Burton, (oak) Tore Hagman;
Fausto Dorelli 6; Paul Forrester: 42-51
inclusive; The Bridgeman Art Library/Getty
Images: 86; John Ittner: 9; Daniele Laberge:
23, 102-3, 143; VHM/DPL/LinkIndia: 91,
MKG/DPL/LinkIndia:125; JM Petit
Publiphoto Diffusion/Science Photo Library:
57; Sam Scott-Hunter: 19, 24-25, 29, 39,
64, 78, 85, 94, and 105.
Other images provided by the authors.*

ARATI

Jaya Jaya Arati Vignavinayaka

Vignavinayaka Sri Ganesha

Jaya Jaya Arati Subramanya

Subramanya Kartikeya

Jaya Jaya Arati Venugopala

Venugopala Venulola

Papavidura Navanita Chora

Jaya Jaya Arati Venkataramana

Venkataramana Sankataharana

Sita Rama Radheshyama

Jaya Jaya Arati Gauri Manohara

Gauri Manohara Bhavani Shankara

Sambasadasiva Uma Maheshwara

Jaya Jaya Arati Raja Rajeshwari

Raja Rajeshwari Tripura Sundari

Maha Lakshmi Maha Saraswati

Maha Kali Maha Shakti

Jaya Jaya Arati Dattatreya

Dattatreya Trimurti Avatara

Jaya Jaya Arati Adityaya

Adityaya Bhaskaraya

Jaya Jaya Arati Shankaraachaarya

Shankaraachaarya Advaita Guruve

Jaya Jaya Arati Sadguru Natha

Sadguru Natha Sivananda

Jaya Jaya Arati Vishnu-devananda

Vishnu-devananda Vishnu-devananda

Jaya Jaya Arati Agastya Munaye

Agastya Munaye Sri Rama Priyaye

Jaya Jaya Arati Ayyappa Swamiye

Ayyappa Swamiye Dharma Shastave

Jaya Jaya Arati Jesus Guruve Moses Guruve, Buddha Guruve

Jaya Jaya Arati Mohammed Guruve Guru Nanak Guruve

Samasta Guru Bhyo Namah

Jaya Jaya Arati Venugopala